MW01235640

PUSH
Labor & Delivery
from the
Inside Out

CATHERINE STACK, N.D., C.N.M.

PUSH
Catherine Stack, N.D., C.N.M.

ISBN: 978-1-07-232825-4

This book is for educational purposes only. It is not
a substitution for medical advice. Please consult
your personal health care providers for your
individual health concerns. Neither Catherine Stack
nor Journey II Health have any responsibility for
any adverse effects arising directly or indirectly as a
result of the information provided in this book.
Trademark names may be used throughout this
book. Rather than put a trademark symbol after
every occurrence of a trademark name, we used
names in an editorial fashion only, and to the
benefit of the trademark owner, with no intention
of infringement of the trademark.

First Printing 2019

DEDICATION

To the babies; past, present and future, who survived the PUSH.

To Mary, the Blessed and Purest Mother of all.

To all current mothers and future mothers-to-be.

PIECES OF US

They take pieces of us.
Our time. Our experience. Our knowledge.
Our gut instinct.
Our mother's intuition.
Our nurse's intuition.
Our motivation and encouragement.
Our focus. Our attention.
Our brazen side, if needed.
Our comic relief.
Those laboring joyfully for their first after years of infertility.
Those laboring for their 6th with their own experience
under their belt.
Those laboring alone with fear in their eyes.
Those laboring for a baby they won't take home.
They all bring a story. They all bring an experience.
They all bring a unique dynamic that only the labor
nurse can sort through and sift out and make head or
tails of to achieve their ultimate goal.
They all bring something.
And they all take.
They all take a piece of us.
Because we will always be a piece of their story.
They own that part of us, in a way.
May we give it like a gift.

Erica Srnsky, RN
Labor and Delivery Nurse ~13 years

CONTENTS

ACKNOWLEDGEMENTS ix
INTRODUCTION xiii

CHAPTER 1
WE ALL JUDGE 21
CHAPTER 2
ADVICE FOR THE MOM-TO-BE 29
CHAPTER 3
DEAR LABOR NURSE 43
CHAPTER 4
THE LABOR COACH 51
CHAPTER 5
ALL IN A DAY 59
CHAPTER 6
BAD THINGS HAPPEN 71
CHAPTER 7
THE BIRTH PLAN 89
CHAPTER 8
STORMS, FULL MOONS & WACKY WEATHER 103
CHAPTER 9
ANATOMY OF A LABOR NURSE 111
CHAPTER 10
HMM…LET'S CLARIFY 123
CHAPTER 11
EPIDURAL OR NOT? 131
CHAPTER 12
HUMOR & BEHIND THE SCENES 139
CHAPTER 13
HAPPY ENDINGS 149
CHAPTER 14
TIME TO PUSH 167

A BABY'S PERSPECTIVE, MAYBE 173

ACKNOWLEDGMENTS

How do you thank 30 years of mentors, co-workers, labor patients and family? To name every person that has been a role model and had an influence on my career as well as my personal life would be a book in itself. So for now, here is a very brief insight into some of the most influential people who have helped to shape the context of this book. They are priceless.

To all of my patients. Your experiences have taught me, humbled me, made me laugh and made me cry. I am not joking when I thank you for letting me be a part of your birth. Most of you are the reason I love my job, and the reason I have met so many wonderful people. Yes, there are a few who make me wonder why I do what I do, but you have also played a very important role. I guess it brings balance and contrast to life.

To Kayla V. Thanks for letting me use this beautiful captured moment for my cover. Your radiance is palpable.

To my retired co-worker, Karen G. Thanks for your permission to use this photo. (And for those who think the baby looks pale, this was within 10 seconds of birth. The cord was not even clamped or cut. I assure you—all was perfect.)

To my sweet Millard Fillmore Hospital co-workers, my work family. You have enriched my life. I love traveling with you, working alongside you, but most of all, I love those priceless moments when we laugh until we start to think it might be time for Depends. Our days are long, but you all make a long day the best it can be. Because of your expertise, my job is easier. I'd work side by side with you any day. It is an honor and I am grateful. I do not forget all of my special friends from Sisters of Charity Hospital and Mt. St. Mary's Hospital. You helped to mold me and lay down a solid foundation as a labor and delivery nurse, and I thank you.

To the Facebook group "Labor & Delivery Nurses Rock!". You have answered questions and provided so much insight, as you are the working core of this amazing specialty. You have taught me that we can be 2000 miles apart and yet so much is the same.

To my children, Josh and Sam. I'm so proud to be your mom and I love when we all get to spend time together—my favorite days. I am so proud of the adults you have grown to be and so glad you still love to spend time with mom and dad.

To Pat, my husband of more than 32 years. Wow, what a ride. Thank you for supporting all that I do, as I know I can be a bit all over the place. We are very different people and it seems to have played out as the perfect formula for a happy life. I am forever grateful and treasure you so deeply.

To Lindsey Wiler, one of the smartest individuals I know. I am grateful for your exceptional talents when it comes to editing, design and keeping me motivated to get this job done. I am constantly in awe of how much you know and can figure out all on your own in such a short period of time. Your ability to be where you are today and still have the time for an old employer is priceless. I love spending time with you. It always equals fun and has made for some amazing memories. This book would not be possible without you and you know it. I am indebted to you for joining me on yet another project.

To my angel friends, guides and protectors from across the veil. It is your support, guidance and nudging that helps me get the job done. Stay with me!

"Appreciation is a wonderful thing: It makes what is excellent in others belong to us as well."

—Voltaire

INTRODUCTION

This book was written for those intrigued by the nuts and bolts of the labor and delivery wing. This is a modern day twist on the popular series "Call the Midwife," hospital style. A variety of readers would benefit from the information in this book. It is my hope that at the end of the read, you will feel like you spent more than a few days interning on our labor wing. I hope you enjoy the experience, as there is something to gain for everyone.

For the seasoned labor and delivery nurse, physician or midwife: You will relate only too well. Good and bad memories will surface. You will laugh. This book will sometimes say what you think, but, due to your professionalism, cannot be said out loud. Your personal experiences will only add richness and depth to this book.

For the new labor and delivery nurse, midwife or intern: You will learn, laugh, and likely be horrified. Please remember, these stories took place over a span of many years. Thousands of uneventful and beautiful deliveries have taken place between the lines of what is disclosed in this book. The extremely wonderful and the horrifically bad experiences are the ones that will become the majority of your memories. All of the beautiful ones in between get blurry and lost in time.

I will compliment and criticize every professional within the system. Within every profession there is the amazing, the average, the bad, and the unfortunate. For the most part, L&D personnel are built tough and I love the vast majority. Many of my co-workers have become family, as we have been through incomprehensible emotional highs and lows. When you experience extreme emotional tragedies or unexplained victories with your co-workers, bonds are formed. This is your work family and you will grow to cherish them.

For the labor support person: You are the husband, partner, wife, mother, friend, doula or entourage that will be witness of and support this amazing event. This book will protect you from anxiety of the unknown. An educated person is much more supportive to someone in labor. You will acquire valuable knowledge that will help you be the pillar of strength to make your loved one's experience the best it can be. You are the ones who will get her through and probably have the most to gain from the insights within this book.

For the critic, especially when it comes to grammar and written language: In order for me to excel at what I do, means that I was probably not so interested in the written and grammatical part of my education. In fact, I bet if there were a high school category, "Least Likely to Write a Book," I may have won. I can barely type without looking at the keys. Something I wish I had paid more attention to such as typing would have come in handy now. So I sit here continuing to peck with two fingers on my keyboard. But this is book number two, and book number one did win a few awards. So, maybe I'm not all that bad. I apologize to the elite in this area, as I am sure I make you cringe at times.

Finally, for the most important, mother-to-be: You will be fascinated by the inner workings of labor and delivery. Some of it may be eye opening, but it is my hope to provide a knowing that brings comfort. Fear of the unknown causes anxiety and stress not worthy of your time and attention. Take a breath, relax, and try to enjoy the experience and unfolding of one of the best days of your life (or at least the meeting of one of the most important people in your life).

After almost 33 years, I am still in love and fascinated by the world of labor and delivery. Then I thought, if I were a mom-to-be, wouldn't I want the inside scoop on this? I don't want the book that fluffs things up or claims that things are supposed to go a certain way. So many women are disappointed that their labor didn't go the way the "book" or "Dr. Google" told them it should go.

If I wanted to become a labor and delivery nurse, midwife or maybe even an obstetrician, wouldn't I want to get a feel for what it is really like? There are many informative books when it comes to labor and delivery, don't get me wrong, but I want to tell the story from the inside out—straightforward, no embellishment. Be prepared, as I will not smooth the rough edges or make it sound glamorous. I am not going to tell every woman that a natural childbirth is the way to go. After all these years I think I have seen almost everything, but I have learned to never let my guard down. The unthinkable can walk through the door at any time. This makes for an interesting and fast read.

For the layperson, experienced or future labor and delivery nurse, OB/GYN, midwife or mom-to-be: I want you to know how different this job is from any other. It's a 2 for 1. Two patients, one chart. You cannot just pay attention to mom—we have a baby to look at as well. This is why emergency room personnel, dentists and even your own medical doctor would like to avoid you until you are all delivered and "normal" again.

I have seen many trainees jump ship, as it is one of the most fast paced, multitasking venues that the medical field has to offer. Ask anyone who works in an urgent care or emergency department. They want that patient with a belly sent to L&D as soon as possible. Pregnant women are weird. They can present so sweet and non-threatening, then—WHAM—shit hits the fan!

We love and hate the adrenaline rush all at the same time. We can't get enough, but are often given too much. We love the unpredictable, yet hate the unpredictable. Labor and delivery people get dirty. We are great multi-taskers, as our brains can work in many directions all at once. L&D nurses are some of the best people I know.

All midwives are not created equal. I have always been comforted by having an extremely competent staff surrounding me. I am a high wire performer with an incredible safety net. I do not need it often, but when I do, I am all too happy it is there. My confidence may actually be somewhat artificial as I know I have excellent support. Take me out of my element, maybe a home birth, I wonder…

So to my home birth and birth center midwife colleagues, I bow to your courage and "knowing" that childbirth is a natural process, your patience and your stamina. I do not think I am built for it but I am glad you are. You are a treasure. I do not have the experience to write your side of the story. I'm sure many of the stories within this book will leave some of you cringing and thinking, "if she would have left that patient alone, that would not have happened." I accept your criticism and probably agree, as hindsight is much more perfect than I.

Unfortunately, there is a disconnect between hospital birth personnel and home birth personnel. The problem is easy to see. As a hospital based employee, we only become witness to home birth when it becomes a problem—such as a 3-day labor that needs a C-section due to fetal distress and maternal exhaustion. The L&D will roll their eyes and think, "Why didn't this person show up 2 days ago?" Or, maybe it presents as a hemorrhage or even fetal death. These things happen, but

I must remind my co-workers that it happens to us as well. This may artificially give home birth a bad name. What we do not see are the hundreds of home births that take place without complication, medication or intervention. We need to remember this.

I am not a very religious person per se, but I am spiritual. I do know that we are not alone. I have had the privilege to witness beautiful miracles. Very often, I feel this profession brings me closer to heaven than church ever did. It is the interaction between humans in this very intense situation that humbles me and lets me know that there is so much more beyond what we see.

It has taken me many years to write this book, but some of the best stories are the ones I have written just out of that raw moment in time. As a nurse or midwife, you typically remember the best of the best or the horrifying worst. Everything in the middle is what ultimately creates the sturdy foundation that makes the amazing and terrifying experiences manageable.

On January 28th 1986, I witnessed my first birth as a young nursing student from Niagara University. I marveled at the labor of this amazing 18-year-old girl who was not far from my own age. The television was on in the room during her labor as a form of distraction. Her labor was going well. At approximately 11:40am, shortly before I was to witness the first birth that would dramatically direct the rest of my life, I witnessed the Space Shuttle Challenger burst into flames. Seven lives were lost in a minute, and one tiny new one was arriving soon. It was a day that would shape the rest of my life.

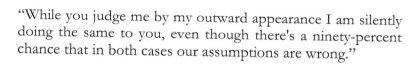

"While you judge me by my outward appearance I am silently doing the same to you, even though there's a ninety-percent chance that in both cases our assumptions are wrong."

—Richelle E. Goodrich

"When we are judging everything, we are learning nothing."

—Steve Maraboli

WE ALL JUDGE
CHAPTER 1

Judging people is something that most of us do unconsciously many times through the course of each and every day. We judge how people look, dress, act, smell. We judge weight, social status and history. We judge educational levels, cars and homes.

When I refer to how we on the labor wing judge our patients, it is not out of rudeness or disrespect, but our own admission to being a human within our specialty.

What we do with judgment is another story. Fortunately, most of the labor and delivery staff are top-notch professionals who are excellent at keeping personal beliefs and opinions to themselves, but every once in awhile I cringe.

When you arrive on the labor wing with your hair done and makeup perfectly applied and tell us you are in painful labor—we judge you and assume we will be sending you home. If you are in labor with your first baby, four centimeters would have you feeling like you could just about die. You cannot walk, talk or focus during strong contractions. So when you arrive all done up, appearing too comfortable for labor, we assume we will be handing your discharge papers after a brief evaluation.

When you feel wet and have had no gush of fluid but say your water is broken, we judge you and beg to differ, especially when it is 95 degrees outside. If you had sex last night and had fluid exit your body the first time out of bed, how is that different from when you are not pregnant? I love to watch sperm swim under the microscope. Typically, when your water breaks, there is an uncontrollable flood that exits through your vagina. It is hard to imagine where all this water is coming from and will continue to keep you wet until the delivery of your baby. Moist or mucous in your underwear are typically not going to get you an admission ticket to the labor and delivery unit. You will also be going home after a brief visit.

When you come in with the complaint of passing your mucous plug, we are confused at what you think we should do about this. Unless you are in labor and/or your water has broken, we don't care much about the mucous plug (unless you are very pre-term). We are confused as to why so much emphasis is placed on it. At the very least, expectant mothers should know that they may notice a glob of mucus weeks to hours before they go into labor, or, not at all.

When you may or may not be in labor and bring a 10-person entourage, we judge you. What are you thinking? We are going to undress you, ask about your history of herpes and genital warts and you really want these people around? Some women have had a history of an abortion that they may prefer to keep confidential—something to think about. But mostly, do you really want all those people looking at your lady parts? I sometimes cringe when the patient's father is in the room while we are checking her, or while she is pushing or giving birth. I don't know about you, but that seems a bit weird to me. I guess I am judging the situation and probably should refrain from doing so.

If you haven't brushed your teeth or bathed in a few days, we take this personally as we know things will get worse. We have to be with you for hours and your body is in for a tremendous amount of work. Good hygiene is not only for your benefit, but is a thoughtful thing to do for the staff that will be caring for you. Many nurses I know will put these patients in the shower before they put them in a bed stating that it will help move the labor along (which is true in many cases). I will reserve judging this patient in a true emergency or an unusually rapid labor.

We judge you based on the doctor you have chosen. Remember, we know these people very well. We basically know what they will order and how they will manage your labor. If this is very different from what you had in mind mind—you just don't know it yet—but we do. Your labor nurse will most likely be your most important advocate if you have landed a physician that practices very differently from your labor expectations and birth plan.

If this is your 10th visit to the labor wing and you think you are in labor again (even though your due date is 3 weeks away), we judge you. We have also gotten to know you by name and you're officially labeled a "frequent flyer." This probably happened after your 3rd visit. "Wannabe" labor patients are frustrating to nurses and doctors alike. We get it. You are tired of being pregnant. Inducing labor so you can get this over with is not in your best interest, nor your baby's. I typically tell my first time mothers, "when in doubt, wait it out." One of two things will most likely happen: contractions will get stronger, or they won't. You should ALWAYS come in if you are not feeling your baby move as he or she normally does.

When you arrive at the hospital, we have trouble with family members who answer all questions for you. You are about to become a mother and we feel you should be perfectly capable of answering your own questions. The exception would be the woman who presents to the labor wing on one cheek, in a wheelchair, and you know that the sounds emanating from her are sounds of pushing. Now we may look to your family for some answers while we get our gloves on.

We judge the length of the birth plan. This is such a hot topic; I have dedicated an entire chapter to it with examples.

We judge you when you have been non-compliant with your prenatal care. When you disregard your blood sugar by showing up drinking an iced cappuccino, or come in smelling like a cigarette factory, we judge you. Our goal is to provide you with an uneventful, uncomplicated birth. By ignoring your own health, you put your baby at risk. These complications often show up in the form of an infant who does not tolerate labor very well. We wonder why you put your baby at risk. We do understand that addictions and habits are hard to break, honestly, but pregnancy should motivate you more than anything else.

As for the mom addicted to pain pills, don't look at us like we are crazy when we say that your baby will go through withdrawal and will most likely have to stay in the hospital for a week or two. The fact that this was not discussed earlier in the pregnancy is unbelievable, but often true. OB/GYN's are rarely experts in narcotic or substance abuse. With the ever-increasing numbers of the addicted population, better education should be made available very early in the pregnancy for staff as well as patients. Most of the time patients addicted to pain pills are poorly educated on what to expect in regard to their newborn, and the side effects are often a blindside.

We will judge you and hide a grin when you are here to have your first baby and say that you do not want anything for pain. You may plan to do things naturally and you are adamant about this. You are typically only 1-2cm at this time and having very mild contractions (you describe them as fairly strong). Hey, we want what you want, but we know that 85% of women will eventually get the epidural, and if you're not okay with that, you will be very disappointed. I have had the experience of working in a hospital that did not offer epidurals. Each and every one of those women survived labor. I know you can do it, but most will opt for an epidural and it's really okay. I applaud the women who deliver without epidurals, I just don't see the need for that intensity level.

If you are a teacher, we judge you. I am sorry to spin this amazing profession to the negative. The exact qualities that make a teacher great in her professional life are the same qualities that make her a nightmare in labor. The typical Type A personality has read all of the books, blogs and websites; she is smart and knowledgeable. The quality she lacks is the "go-with-the-flow" attitude which would make for an easier labor, however, it's just not in her nature. She is very attached to the experience and the outcome she has already formulated in her head. These personality types are more prone to postpartum depression if the experience did not go as planned or if they did not get an A+ according to their own expectations.

If you are a teen, we judge you, but not in the way you may think. I would sign up for this patient each and every time. Their labor is usually quick, easy, and uneventful which makes me think there is something about this age—that maybe they are supposed to have babies. (Stop yelling at me.) This probably would not go over well in this day and age, as many late twenty-somethings are not ready to settle and have a family, my children included. These young mothers are open to an "anything goes" type of birth plan. They tend to trust the process and their caregivers, and the whole experience is just plain easier. When I speak of teens I am referring to the late teen years, 17-19. Anything earlier is unfortunate, but they typically do well from a labor perspective.

If you waited until your early 40's to have a baby, we judge you. Similar to the teacher mentality above, you are typically very educated and in control of almost everything in your life. Please do not take this as an insult. This may be the perfect time for you to have a baby, but labor may be a bit tricky. No fear, we will get you through this.

If you come in on the defense and act as if we will hurt you or your baby... What? We are there to keep you safe. It is our job and our natural human obligation. We will not offer you anything that is unsafe for you or your baby. You must come in with an element of trust. Most labor and delivery nurses are more experienced than your doctor, so this is one of your most important relationships. There must be an element of trust established in order for you to relax and finish your ever important job of child birth.

Now, there are exceptions to everything I have just said. These are just 30 years of generalizations that can't be denied and every seasoned L&D nurse will probably agree.

"I'm not telling you it's going to be easy, I'm telling you it's going to be WORTH IT."

—Art Williams

ADVICE FOR THE MOM-TO-BE
CHAPTER 2

Your nurse is your best advocate and friend. She will get to know you better than your doctor ever does over the course of your labor—trust her. Volume-wise, she's most likely been doing this longer than your doctor. She has lots of experience and will be your best advocate

We know you are scared, but we are here to take care of you. Not only is it our job, but it is within our nature to help others. That's what made most of us choose the healing profession in the first place.

Some of you will read everything that has ever been written about childbirth, consulted with Dr. Google and yet I can tell you, your situation will be uniquely different. As a young, pregnant labor and delivery nurse, I knew I was strong, healthy, and would probably get through without a hitch. I was so sure of this, that I neglected to make my husband take me to birthing classes. A huge mistake on my part, as he was not in any way ready to be a labor coach when things got tough. I could teach him everything he needed to know, right? Wrong.

My water broke at 1:00am in the wee hours of January 11th, just one day past my due date. Back in 1989, especially in smaller hospitals, ultrasounds were typically only done if there was a suspected problem. I did not have one. I did not know the sex of my baby and the due date was calculated based on my regular periods. My contractions started almost immediately, but were not strong and I was excited to be underway. My husband seemed aggravated as I was not in a hurry to get to the hospital, so he took a shower. I know his aggravation was an expression of fear and lack of control or knowledge of the situation. I would get him through it.

What I didn't factor into the equation was by the time I was uncomfortable beyond belief, I could barely get myself through the contractions much less worry about helping my husband get through my labor. No epidurals at this hospital. The best I was going to get was 5mg of Nubain, which is half to one quarter of the dose that is typically given at the hospital I work at now. I knew that Nubain only worked for approximately two hours so I did not want to take it too early.

By 10:00am, I was only 3-4 centimeters and thought I was going to die. The nurses and doctor (my co-workers) kept commenting on how high the baby's head was and not engaging in the pelvis.

Although I was basically a new labor and delivery nurse, I was now a labor patient. Everything I knew went out the window. I was just a girl trying to have her first baby. Just like all moms to be.

I was finally sent to radiology for a CAT scan pelvimetry. In all my years, I have never ever seen this done during labor. I was instructed to hold still while I was positioned flat on my back, not even a pillow. I remember screaming (I'm not a screamer by nature) as the next contraction tore through my body, still not allowed to move. That was not my finest moment and I'm sure the radiology staff was anxious to send me back to the labor wing. I probably scared them to death.

Back to my labor room. My husband is beside himself

and now beginning to act out at the staff as if they are doing something wrong. I cannot care at this moment; I am in too much pain to intervene on anyone's behalf.

Eventually my doctor comes into the room to inform us that I have a rare shaped pelvis type, platypelloid. Only about 5% of women are said to have a platypelloid pelvis. A vaginal delivery is unlikely to happen so I would be scheduled for a cesarean section. Oh thank God, I thought to myself, my husband surely needs a break! (Wink wink.)

I was so happy to end the pain and the light at the end of this painful tunnel was finally in sight. My cesarean was done under general anesthesia so my husband was not allowed in the room. I'm sure he was ecstatic not to be there. When all was said and done, this was the furthest possible experience that I could have conjured up to be my first birth experience. I am not alone and this is not unusual.

At 1:49pm, Joshua Emmett was born weighing 7 pounds 12 ounces. We both did very well. My husband—not so much. He probably suffered a mild form of post traumatic stress disorder.

My second baby, Samantha, was delivered via scheduled cesarean section 21 months later. I was very happy to avoid repeating my previous labor experience. It couldn't have gone any better. Being almost a pound larger, I was even more grateful for my scheduled C-section.

Perspective

It is important to remember that the same scenario given to two different individuals can be perceived in very different ways. Some individuals may have felt as if something went wrong, or someone did something wrong, or something should have been done differently. My experience was different, I admit, but my half full personality tends to keep things positive. The half empty type of personality may feel more like a victim when things don't go as planned.

What type of personality are you? What happens when things do not go as you have intended? Do you tend toward the dramatic type, or go-with-the-flow?

My best advice is to understand that we can all perceive the exact same encounter as very different experiences. Patient perceptions, expectations and fears play a huge role on how the experience will be perceived in the end. If the patient presents to the labor wing with expectations that in her eyes were not met, the experience goes down in her history as a disappointment.

Mira's story is a great example of how perception is not always in line with the actual reality of the situation. I met Mira in my naturopathic practice. She was referred to me for digestive issues. As we got to know each other better, she described to me the birth of her first son. He was born prematurely at 34 weeks, six weeks ahead of schedule. Mira was so disappointed with the outcome. She had to take blood pressure medication and almost had to have a cesarean section. Her little baby boy was born smaller than he should have been at 34 weeks and needed an extended stay in the neonatal intensive care unit. She was so upset about being forced to deliver her baby too early. She feels this was an unnecessary intervention that resulted in his extended stay in the hospital. To this day he is still small for his age, something she feels could have been avoided.

While asking her a few deeper questions, I realized that Mira had suffered from preeclampsia. Preeclampsia is a disorder of pregnancy characterized by the onset of high blood pressure and often a significant amount of protein in the urine. There is usually swelling involved. If left untreated, it could easily escalate to eclampsia, in which life-threatening seizures occur. This is a very basic description of something that could turn catastrophic within hours of onset.

In Mira's case, the fact that her induction of labor went relatively fast tells me that she was truly sick. Inductions for no good reason often take days. In Mira's case, mother nature helped out by expediting the process, which is not unusual when we induce a sick mom. The fact that her tiny baby tolerated the labor is also a testament to his health.

Sometimes the external environment is actually a better place for the baby than the internal environment. This is no fault of Mira's. She actually eats better than 90% of the mothers I know. Sometimes things happen that are out of our control with no rhyme or reason.

Three years after the fact, Mira still feels that she was forced to deliver early, it was unnecessary, and he wasn't ready to be born. She truly feels violated.

My perspective of what she had experienced was to the extreme opposite. In my eyes, it was a great save. Had her blood pressure or preeclampsia gone unnoticed, she may have presented having seizures. Seizures commonly cause oxygen deprivation which could have long term consequences on mom and baby.

The fact that her baby boy had stopped growing suggests that the placenta was no longer doing its job of nourishing her baby. If this were ignored, her baby never would have had the reserve to tolerate labor. She would have most likely been the recipient of a cesarean section due to a fetal intolerance of labor. The worst case would have been a baby that just didn't survive, also known as an intrauterine fetal demise (IUFD).

When I described my perspective to her, it was as if a great weight had been lifted off her shoulders. She really did not understand. Her birth experience was a tragic misperception as she suffered a moderate postpartum depression, which was probably related to her take on things.

To the healthcare provider: please keep in mind that your perspective of a situation can be very different from your patient's. Try to make sure you keep them on the same page as this could be the only difference between a good and bad experience.

Inductions

Inductions of labor are typically done at or after 39 weeks. They can and will be done earlier if medically necessary. Some common reasons include high blood pressure (gestational hypertension), low amniotic fluid level, a baby that is not growing, and more. Most inductions, at least in our institution, are done electively. Elective inductions are done anytime between 39-41 weeks and there need not be a medical reason.

My personal preference is that mother nature knows best and those who come in already in labor have a much faster labor experience. Inductions, especially in first time moms, are a LONG process. This is something I feel is not adequately discussed in the doctor's office at the time it is scheduled. So here comes the patient at 7:00pm, thinking we will magically have her contracting and delivered in a matter of hours. When we gently break it to her and her entourage that she is not likely to have a baby until tomorrow afternoon/evening, the disappointment begins.

With first time moms who have not yet begun to dilate, we usually need to ripen things up with a bit of Cervidil or Cytotec. Both of these ripening agents will hopefully make the Pitocin that follows (maybe 12 hours later), more likely to work. It is not uncommon for these inductions to be a few days before labor begins, or they may even be sent home.

If the cervix has dilated past 2 centimeters and thinned out a bit, this could make all the difference on how fast we will be able to get mom into labor. If it is not her first baby and she has a head start with dilatation, even better.

If I were in the office, scheduling an elective induction, these are conversations I would definitely be having with my patient. I would also state that if the labor wing is busy and there are not enough beds or nurses to safely care for you, your induction WILL be delayed or postponed. When we make these phone calls, the patient who has been delayed is often angry and sometimes even hostile. We understand the disappointment, we really do, but if we have no space for you, there is nothing we can do. To add to that, some of the inductions scheduled for that day ARE medically indicated so the elective inductions go to the bottom of the list. If this were emphasized to the point that mom fully understands, it might not be such a dramatic disappointment when that phone call is made.

I really have nothing against inductions if the cervix is ripe for the inducing or they are medically indicated. I just think moms need to be aware of all of the common scenarios that could take place, including being sent home.

At 39 weeks, most moms would accept the carrot (induction) that is dangled before them in order to end an uncomfortable and long pregnancy. There is nothing wrong with this, we just want you in the know.

More Advice...

If you don't want your child to be medicated or vaccinated, that's okay and you have a right to your opinions and beliefs. But, please do your homework and know what you are talking about before you come in. Have the documentation ready and please tell me that you have discussed this with the doctor you have chosen for your pediatrician. Many people refuse the Vitamin K shot, for example, but really don't know what it's about. Most of us will respect your wishes if you are well informed. Someone who refuses routine care but has not discussed things with their physician or pediatrician is not planning well. You have nine months to do your homework.

Another scenario I see very often is a mom who wants a "natural" childbirth, does not want Pitocin or to have their water broken artificially. This is usually not a big deal or an unusual request—unless you've chosen a physician who practices active management or you have agreed to be induced. Active management is a more aggressive approach to labor that usually involves the addition of Pitocin to give labor a boost and/or breaking the water to "get things going." There is only so much interference that your nurse can run between you and your doctor. Please have these discussions early and repeatedly in your pregnancy.

I have seen active management work well and I have also seen it contribute to a cesarean section. There are valid arguments to both sides of this and there is no right or wrong. The problem lies when you chose a physician that may practice very differently from what you desire.

If you do not want an episiotomy, have this discussion prior to coming to the labor wing. The earlier, the better. Fortunately, episiotomies are becoming less and less routine, but there still doctors out there that will do one every single time. The good news: doctors are getting their hands slapped for doing them. Our hospital keeps track of who's doing them. There is a time and place for episiotomy, but in most cases, it is unnecessary and actually precipitates the need for more suturing (stitches).

Ask around. Ask nurses, ask other moms, or call the labor wing of the hospital where you plan to deliver. There may be the hard-ass nurse who pretends she cannot give you that information, so call again. Most of us would be happy to make a recommendation based on what you are looking for and where you live. Really, it would make our job easier if you were aligned with the doctor that practices what you are looking for.

Here is a fairly common scenario I want you to consider: you are now 41 weeks. You have done a great job and are very proud of yourself for not caving into your doctors offer for induction. You are going "natural" and want no intervention. Your water breaks. You are initially excited. FINALLY you will be going into labor, or so you think. Eight hours later—nothing. Now you arrive at the hospital 1 centimeter dilated, 50% effaced (thinned out) and -2 station. Your body still hasn't gotten the memo that it's time to go into labor. This scenario typically ends in a 2-3 day labor, an exhausted mom, and an increased risk for postpartum depression. Would you consent to an induction (Cervidil or Cytotec) if this were you in order to avoid a 2-3 day scenario? I would. Very few moms-to-be factor in the loss of sleep and inevitable fatigue after an extended labor experience. Again, most of us support whatever it is you want, but it hurts our hearts that you think you always have to take the long hard road to consider yourself successful.

Some of Your Complaints...Valid to Ridiculous!

The following comments were anonymous patient survey comments collected from two different hospitals. Most of the comments are very complimentary and even mention the staff member(s) names. This does come back to us and we appreciate it more than you could ever know. It makes us glad to have chosen this profession. Many of the complaints were similar, even though the hospitals differed by location (suburban and inner city). I will add my own two cents for your reading pleasure. Don't worry, I will call the staff out as well in another chapter.

"It would have been nice to have control of the Heat/AC in my room."—We agree! This is a common battle within the staff. The menopausal, hot flashing nurses usually win. The rest of us wear fleece. Since the initial writing of this, we now have individual controls in each labor room.

"Air vent in ceiling too loud."—Consider it white noise. Really? I would never think to complain about this. I think some individuals feel the need to find something to complain about.

"Most nurses were excellent. I only had 2 nurses that were not very attentive and one wouldn't give me my pain meds 12 hours after my C-section."—If this is actually true, it is appalling. My advice to anyone who feels they are being ignored or mistreated is to call the charge nurse or hospital switchboard and request to page the nursing supervisor to your room. That will have a second set of eyes looking at you almost instantly. Don't be mean, just explain the situation to the supervisor and things will get taken care of quickly.

"All nurses were pleasant and helpful but seemed very understaffed and spread thin."—We actually don't mind this type of complaint. We can only hope they will add more staff. Unfortunately, there are just those days where no number of people can accommodate the volume that walks through our doors. We will always do our best.

"This section is difficult for me to rate. I had very good

37

experiences with everyone on staff except for one night nurse on the maternity unit. Her name was_____ and she was horrible, very curt, mean, not helpful. I complained and the charge nurse took care of me for the rest of the night."—GOOD GIRL!!! Speak up! I have no problem with you calling people out by their name. I wish more people would. There have likely been other complaints about this nurse. Unfortunately, the union protects these people. In my perfect hospital, it would be three strikes and you're out policy.

"Nurse who started my IV missed 3 times before successfully starting it. I had three bruises as a result."—Are you overweight? Dehydrated? Generally a difficult stick? Most labor and delivery nurses are excellent at starting IV's. They do it all the time and you are not likely to find nurses better than L&D or ER nurses when it comes to IV's. Most nurses will try twice then call for help before the third stick. We have even called the anesthesiologist for our more difficult patients. Sometimes it is not our fault.

"There were not enough chairs in the labor room for my visitors." —Really? Do you enjoy having people start at you while you are in labor? Most labor nurses have enough trouble keeping the IV tubing, monitor cords and plugs from strangulating you and tripping her. We have no control over the size of the room. We do need to have the room ready to move fast and get to the sink to wash our hands. I know you want us to wash our hands. The more chairs that clog the room, the more our job becomes difficult which ultimately affects you. Let your visitors come stare at you at home.

"Everyone wore strong perfume. It should not be allowed"—I would probably disagree with this statement as it is highly unlikely that the staff member is wearing a strong cologne. The majority of people who are overly sensitive to smells typically have a chronic and deep rooted gastrointestinal issue. They usually have a growing allergy list as well and maybe even allergic to latex. If this is you, I highly recommend a cleanse after you deliver and maybe even probiotics.

These are just some of the comments taken from our

discharge evaluation forms. These do not represent the hundreds of personal letters and pictures of gratitude and thanks that make our hearts swell. These letters are what sometimes get us through the most difficult days.

So are you ready, mom-to-be? We are ready for you. It is okay to be afraid, we know you have never done this before and even if you have, each experience is different. Trust us, trust your doctor but most of all, trust your body and gut instinct as it typically knows what to do.

"As a nurse we have the opportunity to heal the mind, soul, heart and body of our patients, their families and ourselves. They may forget your name, but they will never forget how you made them feel."

—Maya Angelou

DEAR LABOR NURSE
CHAPTER 3

Insider Tips for the Labor Nurse

I probably have very little advice to offer the seasoned labor nurse. My intuition, senses and skills have evolved and been enhanced by most of them.

Becoming a labor and delivery nurse is exciting as well as scary as hell. I remember way back when I didn't think I would ever be able to tell how dilated someone was. It all felt mushy "in there" to me. Timing everything was extremely stressful as well. If you called the OB doctor in for delivery too early you couldn't miss the scowl or growl directed your way. Most doctors would love to enter the room with just enough time to wash their hands and glove up and deliver the baby on the second push from entering the room.

As a new nurse, the horrifying thought of not having the doctor in the room when the patient delivers keeps you calling them in early, sometimes for years. This is a very common situation for the newbie. Eventually, it will happen. That baby will come so fast when it is just you, mom and dad. And guess what? Everyone will be fine, including you. The most important thing you could ever learn is to hide the panic or fear. Patients will sense this. If you are calm, they will remain calm. This is initially hard as there are so many things to think about when caring for your labor patient.

As a new nurse, you are going to over-analyze strips, under-analyze strips, and miss cues you shouldn't have missed. You will not be comfortable in your skin for a few years. Competent? Yes. Comfortable? No. This may be longer or shorter depending on the volume of patients your hospital delivers over the course of the month. If you are in a hospital that delivers under 50 babies per month, as I once worked at, it will take longer for you to find your experience and your comfort. The upside to this is that you do not typically have a whole team around you to help when things get crazy. This will help sharpen your skills in no time and you will actually come to learn and do more than labor and delivery nurses in larger institutions, because you are often the only one there.

First babies are no speed demons when it comes to delivery. Although there is always the exception, the first 5 centimeters take forever, and then 5-10 centimeters will typically pick up the pace a bit. Moms will work the hardest to get this one out. If they have an epidural, let that head come down or "labor down" to a +1 or +2 station before you even think about pushing. The station of the head is determined by specific anatomical points in the pelvis, the ischial spines. Another learned skill in the world of labor and delivery. If you push as soon as she is fully dilated and that head is higher than a zero station like -1 or -2, you will likely push at least 1.5 to 2 hours, or longer. If you wait until the head comes down to a +2 station, you will most likely push less than 1 hour. This is one of the perks that come with an epidural. You are not changing the time of delivery by much, but you are preventing an overly exhausted mom and a higher risk for forceps or vacuum assisted delivery. I wish those who fear or oppose epidurals would really make a note of this point. This would be a great time to utilize the peanut ball, especially if the baby is in the occiput posterior position. Occiput posterior is a baby facing the wrong direction which leads to painful back labor and a possible prolonged labor. This device literally looks like a giant Mr. Peanut that will be placed between mom's legs in a side lying position. An excellent L&D nurse will assist mom in changing her position frequently in order to facilitate head descent.

For the mom who does not want an epidural, she will tell you when she is pushing. You will have little say. If she has the urge and is fully dilated, let her push. Women who don't have epidurals will do much better if they stay out of the bed. Walking, birthing balls, squatting and warm showers will help keep her engaged and motivated.

Never trust second babies. This is the child that will most likely be the shortest labor for moms. They will be 4 centimeters one minute and fully dilated the next. If this mom wants an epidural please do not hold her off as long as possible. She is likely to miss her window of opportunity and although some may be empowered by this, most will be angry. You will not have done her any favors. Remember, it is not your pain or experience to judge. If she knows she wants an epidural, it is much harder to sit through one at 8 centimeters than it is at 5 or 6 centimeters. I'd be calling her doctor in when she is 8 centimeters if she does not have an epidural. If she is comfortable with an epidural, you have more time. Be wary of pushing with a mom having her second, third or fourth baby. The power of just one push can have her crowning and you will be scrambling in order to get things ready and people in place.

Moms having their third baby will typically have a labor duration that falls between their first and second labors. I don't think I have ever read this anywhere, but after a whole bunch of years, it is a valid generalization.

The one phrase I want you to pay very close attention to is when your mom in labor says, "the baby is coming." Listen to her. You will not usually hear these words from the first time mom. This is much more common in the woman who has done this a time or two.

A pet peeve of mine is when I overhear a nurse say to a patient something like, "Why didn't your doctor or nurse do this or that?" or "They should have done ____." This places the negative notion that something was not done right. Ugh. Now I know I've got some damage control in reestablishing trust as this well meaning nurse just put some doubt in the patient's head that maybe something should have been done differently. Sometimes this is not far from the truth as hindsight is always much more accurate, but it does absolutely nothing as far as making that patient feel comfortable and safe.

My advice to all labor nurses: keep your difference of opinion out of your patient's room. Right or wrong, it creates doubt in their mind that will never serve you well, even if you are right. I have often heard birth stories from women that are amazingly distorted and fabricated (I know this—I was there). Do not add fuel to that fire! In a world of excessive litigation, keep that patient's environment safe and secure. If I polled the patient, her husband, the mother and the nurse about the particular labor experience, you'd be surprised at the different perspectives of the same delivery. From the labor staff perspective, it was a perfect delivery. Then you later find out that the patient's interpretation was far from perfect. Be careful. Being a good communicator is essential when caring for others. So many experiences can get lost and misinterpreted in what was not communicated correctly.

One of the best pieces of advice I have ever heard was from a physician turned attorney giving a lecture on OB litigation. He stated that very few people can assess or evaluate a health care provider's competence, but most will hold you accountable based on your compassion or lack of. Many lawsuits have nothing to do with competence. Unfortunately, we are not always able to provide a perfect outcome but we can be very compassionate to the situation. Compassionate people rarely find themselves in a lawsuit.

There is no excuse for a mean nurse. Your bad day, home life or a busy labor wing are all invalid excuses. Hospitals would improve quality in care if they initiated a "3 strike, you're out" policy when it comes to hospital staff. Yes, some patients are very difficult, rude and demanding. But with a little tact, you can come out a winner without being labeled as mean. This is the one area that I feel the union protects the bad guy. There are amazing nurses and nursing students out there who are kind, compassionate and would love and deserve to take the job of a cranky nurse.

There is a right and a wrong way in dealing with even the most difficult patient. What we have to remember, as we often forget, is that people are not themselves when they are scared. Think about it. Once someone is more comfortable, there is usually a change in personality as they begin to let their guard down.

I rarely have trouble getting along with even the most difficult personality. But on this one occasion, I just couldn't make this patient happy. Her mother was overly loud at how unhappy they were about the care of her daughter. I could do no right. She was too hot, too cold, the IV hurt, the pain wasn't being properly managed and so on. This makes for a very draining day. Then a light bulb went off in my head. I knew there was more to their misery than me—I was just the unfortunate target of the moment. This is how I resolved the issue without getting defensive or rude.

Our unit usually has an intern (first year resident) and a midwife to manage labor. Typically, the midwife has many more years of experience and is far more skilled. This is in no way meant to be insulting or question the competence of the first year intern, it is just a matter of experience.

So into the patient's room I went. I proceeded to sit on the corner of her bed and said, "I know you are not happy with the care you are receiving. Even though I can only do my best with the 30 years of experience that I have, sometimes people just don't have good chemistry. So to help you out, I will be turning over your care to our new first year intern, who is anxious to learn all she can. She is younger and you will love her!" With that, there was a gasp from the mother and a very extreme change of mood and atmosphere. The patient apologized and ask if I would continue to care for her. "Are you sure?" I asked. The rest of the visit went well and there were no repercussions or bad reviews.

Nurses could do the same thing by stating that we have a new labor nurse who would love the experience and I'd be happy to switch assignments with her. Typically, a good charge nurse will help rearrange assignments for you. There will be times that this is not possible and you are just going to have to stick out the rest of that shift. You WILL get through it no matter how draining it is. Remember, this is a very small minority of all the patients you will care for.

Caring for friends and family is a tricky situation. This often becomes a very mixed bag of experiences and emotions. It has been my experience that things don't often go as planned and this is a scenario that makes us feel a bit more helpless than we typically do. We know this woman and want her to have the exact labor she has been expecting. The labor nurse inside of us tries to remain objective and focused but the friend/family side tends to feel a bit more unstable when things take a turn for the unpredictable. This will be the patient you miss the IV on when you have had no trouble with the last twenty you have started. In a nutshell, it tends to be more uncomfortable. I'm not suggesting you refuse to care for family and friends, just know it may be a bit more taxing than you expect. It is hard to stay objective with people you have outside relationships with.

A special note for the MOM-TO-BE readers of this book, do not fret. Obstetrical nurses will get you through your labor and delivery experience typically without a hitch. The majority of labor and delivery nurses LOVE their jobs and will do everything to help you have the best experience possible. Be sure to ask questions when you have them. Communication goes both ways and is a very important tool when it comes to making the most of your birth experience.

"Surround yourself with people who support you. Find champions."

—Sarah Gavron

THE LABOR COACH
CHAPTER 4

The labor coach is a pivotal part of the labor experience. They come in all shapes and sizes. They are mostly FOB's (father of the baby), but sometimes they are a friend, partner, a mother, a sister or a whole group of people. Some moms will hire a doula.

Back in the day, fathers were not even allowed in the delivery room. The famous scenario in many of our heads was a dad pacing in the waiting room and eventually handing out cigars when the news finally came of a boy or a girl. Gross! I guess I am old enough to remember smoking at the nurses' station (OMG), starting IV's without gloves, and even being handed a newborn baby without gloves. I'm still alive—amazing! But when you think about all the new and "right" ways to raise a baby, I am also surprised my children survived childhood. I had bumper pads on the crib, they had blankets and stuffed animals. My children had pacifiers and walkers with wheels. They slept on their tummies. I'm not sure how I raised two very well adjusted children, now adults, when according to today's recommendations, I did most things wrong.

Things have certainly changed and mostly for the better when it comes to the labor coach. My husband might disagree, as he was one of the few who did not want to see any of it. He actually did not do well with seeing me in pain. If I were the labor nurse for my own birth, I would not have liked the way my husband acted and reacted to something that went fairly normal. I always try to remember this. I take some responsibility for this since I did not make him go to classes. After all, I was a labor nurse (brand new), I could walk him through this. NOT. Go to the classes, if not for yourself, do it for your labor coach. You do not want them to panic as your head spins and words you have never before spoken come flying out of your mouth. Foul outbursts happen far less than rumor has it, but when you are in indescribable pain, you are in no mood or shape to comfort and educate your labor coach.

The most bizarre experience I had with labor coaches was when I had the current boyfriend holding one leg while the father of the baby was holding the other leg as she pushed. This actually went well. Weird, but well.

A similar story did not go so well. Both possible fathers were present for the delivery. The actual paternity was unknown, but mom had it narrowed down to two prime candidates (I am still shaking my head on this one). These labor coaches spent much of their time sleeping. Our mom-to-be had better support from her own mother and one of the potential grandmothers. Now I was not actually in on this delivery, but I do recall one of the "baby daddy" candidates storming out of the room after delivery, his mom in toe, saying that the baby did not look like him. Really? This could have been a Jerry Springer episode.

One of the more awkward experiences was caring for a seemingly happily married couple expecting their third child. The labor went well, he was an attentive and supportive coach. She was sweet, had an epidural and all went textbook perfect. The baby's head began to crown. (Crowning occurs when we can see the baby's head through the thinning and stretching vagina and perineum. This typically lets us know delivery is imminent.) Funny thing about this baby was that I had two fair haired parents and this baby seemed to have kinky dark hair, but I did not think much of it until this little one was born.

This baby boy actually looked African American. Hmm. When black babies are born, they are typically pale looking but the giveaway details are that kinky cute hair and the very dark scrotum or vulva (reproductive parts). So now everyone of the delivery staff is acknowledging this without saying a word. I'm not sure if the parents are aware of anything out of the norm, but are happy and celebrating. It is truly none of our business, but wow, inquisitive minds would surely like an explanation for this or maybe all is better left unsaid.

Stereotypes
Here are some classic labor coach stereotypes. Most L&D personnel would agree, I checked.

The Sleeper: We have to crawl over you to get to your wife. You don't budge or move when we come into the room. And for some strange reason, your laboring wife does not seem to mind.

The Controller: Answers all questions. This is probably the most annoying for a nurse. Unless she is unconscious or pushing, the mother of your baby is fully capable of answering her own questions—so zip it!

The Lovey-Dovey: This is the coach who is constantly touching or kissing his wife in labor. Eventually, we hide a smile when she turns to him and screams, "Stop touching me!" Poor thing. He is trying but labor is not the time for smothering behaviors.

Panicked: This is the coach who you would really like to remove from the room. Their fear is infectious. It is a distraction that sets the stage for an uncomfortable experience.

The Fainter: This happened with much more frequency when we used to allow dads to stay in for the epidural procedure. We don't anymore. I would bet that most readers would assume a fainting father happens more often than it actually does. I've had a dad or two slide down my body as I attempt to hold his wife's leg while the doctor applies a vacuum or forceps, but an alert labor nurse will usually see it coming before they go down. We have sent a dad or two down to the emergency department for a bump on the head as they went down faster than we could intervene. If dad is on his way out, he will typically lose all color in his face and you notice that he is feeling a bit warm and might be removing his outer clothing. The experienced labor staff will see this and make sure he immediately goes to a sitting position. A helpful staff member will usually arrive with a cup of juice that will help him perk back up in no time.

The Perfect One: The best coach ever. Not too gushy not too distant, keeps calm under pressure, and provides great support for his wife. Nurses will fall for this guy, but not to worry mom, he is ultimately into you and this amazing experience.

Mr. Angry and Pissed to be There: Does not trust the staff and is totally convinced that the mother of his baby is not getting the best care. He really does not act that into her either. He is alienating the staff and ultimately affecting his wife's experience. We wish he would have been left home.

The Worry Wart: He will question everything. Has a hard time understanding that this is not your first rodeo. This may intimidate the new labor nurse, but the seasoned nurse will only smile and sometimes even deliver a few good comebacks.

The Wannabe Obstetrician: Put some gloves on this guy and let him help you catch. This is typically a fun delivery. He can't seem to get his face out of the way of the impending birth. If all is going well, this is the perfect candidate for a birth assistant. He will talk about it for the rest of his life.

The Eater: Foods that smell and bags of candy line the counter tops. The room is full of wrappers and old food smells that would make even a non-laboring person vomit.

The Techie: He has his computer, camcorder, long lens camera and chargers for all. He's got the HDMI cables in order to watch Netflix on the hospital television. He comes prepared, but when it comes to that moment of birth, he forgets to take pictures and barely remembers how to turn the camera on. A good labor nurse will help the poor guy as his intentions were so good.

Doula or Don't?

A doula, also known as a birth companion or post-birth supporter, is a non-medical person who assists a woman before, during or after childbirth, along with her spouse and family, by providing physical assistance and emotional support.

I have mixed feelings about doulas on the labor wing. If the mom-to-be desires no epidural, then they are well placed as this mom needs lots of support to get through all the stages of labor. This is very important. They need to have the experience and confidence to be able to get mom (and dad) through some pretty intense situations if they know what they are doing. This doula is the one that the labor & delivery staff truly appreciates as we know how hard it is to keep mom focused and panic-free.

If the mom-to-be thinks she will end up with an epidural, my best advice is to leave the doulas to prenatal education, and more importantly, postpartum and breastfeeding care. I feel mothers could benefit from an earlier discharge if they had a doula in place to help the first few days to a week. Healthcare costs could be dramatically reduced when it comes to childbirth, as early discharge could be an option.

Going home with a brand new baby is probably one of the most stressful parts of childbirth. The reality of responsibility hits you in the face with an intensity you would have never expected, nor have you prepared for as you were so focused on the childbirth portion of this event. It is in the first few days that I would have appreciated a check-in by someone who knew what they were doing. All the labor and delivery experience did not in any way prepare or comfort me when it came to taking my first newborn home. I was scared to death.

Most labor coaches do a great job. Childbirth is an amazing process and it is so easy to become actively engaged in the experience. Moms would be wise to choose a person who calms them, makes them laugh and truly enjoys their company. Every once in a while, the father of the baby is not the best candidate.

My best advice is to leave people home that tend to be anxious or dramatic. These individuals will serve no functional purpose in your labor experience. If it's too late and these individuals have made their way into you labor experience, use your labor nurse to help remove them. This way there are no awkward feelings between you and said individual. You will have to see them again, we don't.

"The problem is that those of us who are lucky enough to do work that we love are sometimes cursed with too damn much of it."

—Terry Gross

ALL IN A DAY
CHAPTER 5

Sometimes, running the labor wing feels comparable to conducting an orchestra, not that I ever have, but you are trying to organize multiple layers of people to be at the right place at precisely the right time. Doctors need to be kept up to date, patients need to be checked, and anesthesia on call for epidurals and possible cesarean sections. Nurses can hopefully be one on one with their active labor patients (which are actually two patients in one), but often, they have two moms as the labor wing volume has no rhyme or reason. Just like the emergency department, we have no idea what will walk around the corner at any given time. There is no predictability, aside from full moons and weather events, which all who work in the realms of medicine would attest to.

Then we have the already delivered moms, all done and getting to know their new babies while creating a log jam in which space becomes a premium. This happens often. The labor wing staff must get very creative—you ALWAYS want a room available. Moms are entitled to their two-day stay (three for cesarean sections) as there is much teaching that takes place. I find irony in the length of stay for these patients. Open heart recipients can go home in as little as three days. Major surgeries can go home the same day. However, normal vaginal deliveries get two days. This is weird to me. This is where I feel doula's or Home Health Aides would serve a cost effective purpose. I digress, back to my day.

My drive to work is about 45 minutes and I am up at 4:45am. I hate to be rushed in the morning, cherish that first cup of coffee, and love a hot shower.

6:40am. I'm on deck and ready to roll. I'm on the lookout for my fellow midwife as I'm sure she is ready to abandon ship, since we obviously could use a bigger boat today.

I used to work 12 hour nights and often don't even remember how I got home some nights. The divots on the side of the road have saved me more than once. They give your body a surge of adrenaline for having almost fallen asleep behind the wheel. Chewing ice also seemed to work well for me. A funny remedy for another night nurse was putting her hair in the window so if she were to doze her hair would get pulled. Ouch, but I get it.

Nine full birthing rooms. Monitors chiming everywhere, uncontrolled sounds of pushing that obviously weren't expected, as everyone goes scrambling into the room that was not prepared for an imminent delivery. Chris, our lovely night shift midwife is ending her shift with a bang. Gloved and ready to deliver a little one who just didn't want to wait until we were ready or her doctor was here. I ask if I can relieve her but she stays to finish as I leave the room to attempt to make some sense of a labor wing that has apparently gone mad.

Just trying to catch up with what's going on and keeping progress notes up to date as you are being called in five different directions at once can definitely be overwhelming to even the most experienced team.

7:05am. Mindy arrives. A very sweet woman from Afghanistan. She has recently moved from California to Buffalo. I always wonder how people from warmer climates can survive here. It is a great place summer and fall, but those long winters…

Mindy is only 35 weeks and is complaining that she is bleeding. She is not uncomfortable but is very concerned that she has nothing ready for the baby. After a gentle exam, I inform her that she is 4 centimeters and has a bit of bloody show and that she is in labor. Now she is afraid that it is too early for her baby. I reassure her that even if he needs a little help, all will go well. Mother Nature tends to know when the baby will be better off outside the body and this is when preterm labor happens. I now need to figure out where we will put her.

7:15am. Chris is ready to give me reports and fill in the missing pieces that I have begun to figure out with the help of the nursing staff. I know her night was rough and she also has a long drive home. I don't know how she does it.

7:30am. Caroline is in room 9. Her labor is progressing well and I examine her and find her to be 9 centimeters. I can only feel a bit of cervix so I am assuming she will be fully dilated shortly. Due to the business of the labor wing, I give her doctor a call suggesting that she should head in. Most physicians are very easy to work with, but there are a few that seem to do their very best in making you feel that you're bothering them or crying wolf. On this very busy day, she reminded me that she only lives four minutes from the hospital. Geeze, if only I had the time to check her patient every 10 minutes so I could inform her when it was the exact time to come, in order for her to not miss the delivery. It is not in my nature to have to rush in for a delivery; having notice, I would think, is the considerate measure. Not this physician. She told me to call her when the baby's head was crowning (essentially, when you can see the baby's head at the vaginal opening). WHAT? I was more than a bit disgusted, but knew her patient was in excellent hands. Needless to say, we did call her when the baby was crowning and I proceeded to deliver a beautiful baby girl quite easily at approximately 8:00am. I never mind this; it is one of the best parts of my job.

I typically work with an intern and by this time of year, which is May, they are soon to be in their second year and typically have the basics down. Sundays, for whatever reason, we do not have an intern. Today is Sunday. I do however, have a second or third year resident to scrub on a cesarean section if the occasion arises, but they hate coming to the labor wing. It's as if they have done their time on the labor and delivery deck. My favorite part of women's health is labor. It is action packed.

Having just worked the previous day, I had some prior knowing as to what would be the flavor of the day—busy. Two inductions, at least one or two of the women I had yesterday would be undelivered, and whatever else might walk through our doors. A bit busy for a holiday weekend Sunday, but I happen to work with some of the best nurses and know we will get through anything.

We always have an in-house attendant who is typically a well seasoned OB/GYN. A rare few leave you praying that nothing bad happens so you do not have to call them. Most of the time they willingly keep checking in to make sure you are okay, but for some, you will only see their faces when they hand off their pagers to their relief. This is not as bad as it sounds. It just means we did a great job, and our busy labor wing was uneventful.

On my weekends, I like to bring or make a healthy breakfast since our cafeteria is closed until lunch. That leaves us to a coffee and doughnut shop which serves little purpose when it comes to the nutrition needed to sustain you over a 12.5-hour shift. I am always in awe over hospital food. You would think the hospital would want wounds to heal quickly, blood sugar to be stabilized, and toxicities to be cleaned out, not put in. You'd think that a hospital would want to minimize disabilities in their staff and reduce call-ins. One would assume that a teaching hospital would teach people to eat in order to minimize illness. This is not the case. Ice cream, sherbet, bread, mashed potatoes, breaded chicken and diet soda are just some favorites. God help the healthy eater! There are no raw foods or fresh juices to be found anywhere. If you ask for a salad, you are likely to get a few small pieces of iceberg lettuce, four shreds of a carrot and a cherry tomato. Then add the chemical loaded salad dressing—just shoot me! I once questioned the sickly head of the dietary department. Her response was that people want french fries and ice cream. I give up.

Back to the labor wing. On this particular day I was going to be behind the eight ball when it came to eating anything. I hate that. I need my food!

Three other labor patients were progressing well and their babies were behaving. There isn't much more for me to do besides make sure things stay well and keep their physicians informed. One of the inductions had been admitted two nights prior. Poor thing. Sara was 39 weeks but had a few common complications that indicated that delivery would be best prior to the due date. I wished that Mother Nature would have received the memo. Things tend to go much better when she does. Gestational diabetes and hypertension are risk factors that may complicate the health of the baby or complicate the delivery. When we need to induce a mom for these reasons, it would be reasonable to inform her that this could take days to get her into labor. If we informed them from the beginning, it would not feel like torture when day one and two slide by without a baby. The other side to this is the mom who is really sick with preeclampsia or eclampsia (seizures) or something known as HELLP Syndrome. These women tend to deliver very fast once the induction is initiated, as Mother Nature is on the same page. I am always in awe, the body knows.

For the record, inductions are long. If your cervix is not at least dilated to 2-4 centimeters, plan on a long stay before labor even begins. Spontaneous labor is much quicker and typically uncomplicated. When I question one of my new admissions, she tells me her first labor was 36 hours. The actual story usually is that it took 20 hours to get her into labor and the remaining 16 are normal for a first baby.

Sara had recently received an epidural after about 30 hours of trying to get her into labor. They had broken her water during the night in hopes of moving things along. Little progress was made (but at least she slept) and my morning sign-out was looking a bit gloomy in regards to a vaginal birth. Fortunately, Sara's doctor was patient and as long as mom and baby showed no signs of distress, she would let us continue to change positions and ride this out.

10:30am. A gravida 8 para 4 arrives with ruptured membranes in labor. Gravida means how many times a woman has been pregnant, para (which can be further broken down) essentially means how many births/children. Because she's had two previous cesarean sections, I will need to hurry and get her admitted for her third as she did not want to labor at all. The resident sees I am drowning but does little to help me admit this patient. I finally get it done at 5:30pm that evening, long after the baby was delivered by cesarean section.

Another mom-to-be, Kelly, also arrived late morning. I had seen her once before, approximately 4 weeks prior, when she was dropped off by her drug addicted and abusive boyfriend. He would not come back to get her and left her to sit. We do have information that we give when we suspect abuse, but we can't force these women to do anything about it. Here she is now, back for her induction, and the supposed FOB (father-of-baby) wanted a paternity test because he wasn't taking a care of "any f-ing baby that wasn't his." What a piece of garbage. He did not want the baby to have his name, but only told me that outside the room so he didn't make her cry. What a stellar citizen. Well no worries there, as we always have the mom and baby under the same name. They are the ones filling out the birth certificate a day or two later. One minute he is yelling at her, and one minute kissing her tired and laboring leg. So bizarre. He said if the baby is Mexican or black then we know for sure, but if it's a white baby, he wants paternity test. I ask him why this is coming up now, and inform him that we do not do paternity tests without a court order. Most will get it done via a pediatrician order. If it were not his baby, he would put her out on the street. In all my years, I have never witnessed such a complete jerk. His mom called from out of state to talk to me. I did not want to hear her story, nor could I provide her with any information. She wanted to make sure her son's name was not listed on the birth certificate. My only comment was that this was an extreme case and social workers would be getting involved. I feared for Kelly and her baby. I still feel I will read about them at some point.

Back to Sara. It is now approximately 1:00pm and we have not stopped. Poor Sara has been here for two days. Her doctor was on the labor wing taking care of some charting, when from her room comes a blood curdling scream. A moment later, I deliver her baby, gloveless and unprepared. Her doctor walked in the room a moment later, stunned, as we all were, that after all this time, she missed the delivery. Mom and baby did very well.

Mary is a healthy 42-year-old having her first baby. She has the body of a 20-year-old which has me in awe. Her labor has gone well, but now she is pushing for almost 3 hours. That is hard to watch.

1:30pm. Lucy, a 28-year-old G4 P2012 (4th pregnancy, 2 full term deliveries, 0 preterm deliveries, 1 miscarriage, and 2 living children) presents at 35 weeks, complains that she covered her pee hole, then covered her vag hole, and was more wet from the vag hole. I assure you, I could not think to make this up. I notice that her makeup is perfectly applied as she informed me that she was an LPN (licensed practical nurse). Oh, and one little detail she didn't mention was a stroke she suffered nine months ago. WHAT? She received TPA (a drug used in stroke victims to help dissolve clots) and suffered speech difficulty and right sided weakness. She was in rehab for 6 weeks. I'm trying to swallow this information rather than throw-up. "Who's your neurologist?" I ask. She has not seen anyone since December, and it is now May. WHAT? "Who is your medical doctor?" I ask. She informs me that his office closed in January. WHAT? "Are you on any medications, such as blood thinners, that would reduce potential complications?" She replies, "No, I took myself off when I found out I was pregnant." WHAT? Now I am going to be sick. Lucy is approximately 350 pounds. I questioned her about blood sugar. Her doctor said she was borderline diabetic but continues to describe many symptoms that make me think hypoglycemia or SVT (supraventricular tachycardia). Yup, she had that too. This girl was a time bomb that had fallen through the cracks. By this time, I was the one having shortness of breath and heart palpitations. Six hours to go.

After all was said and done, Lucy's water had not broken and she was not dilated. That's great because I could not wait to send her home. I left a long note with her OB/GYN, who I am sure will implement a plan to deliver the baby when Lucy is ready in 4-5 weeks. Did I mention she had a placenta that was partially covering her cervix? Just another potentially life threatening complication.

5:00pm. A 42-year-old, non-English speaking Russian woman having her ninth baby was sent in for evaluation of blood pressure. Her blood pressure ranged from 170/ 97 to 187/114. For those of you with no medical background, these are extremely high blood pressures that could very easily result in in a seizure, stroke for mom, and or a placental abruption. A placental abruption is when the placenta literally separates from the uterine wall. A complete separation would result in the death of the baby and possibly a life threatening hemorrhage for mom. Both would be very scary scenarios that could result in the death of mom, baby, or both. She was 36 weeks along and an induction of labor is indicated. She's had eight previous vaginal births without difficulty and this little 36-week-old should be fine. After getting a detailed history with the help of a translator phone, the admission is complete and medications are initiated to help us control and bring down her blood pressure.

This was, I'm sure, a very scary event for this mom. The language barrier alone is extremely stressful. I have delivered many mothers who do not speak English and for the most part, the language of labor is universal and we get by just fine. In this case, she refused the induction. She felt that she was putting her baby at risk by delivering early. After 45 more minutes on the phone with our Russian interpreter, she was still not ready to move forward with the induction. The medication was finally beginning to stabilize blood pressure, but this was still a very scary situation for all involved. Her bloodwork suggested that this was not preeclampsia.

The next day, this patient wanted to leave the hospital against medical advice (AMA). The medications are working to keep her blood pressure in a safe range. She has every right to refuse medical treatment and leave the hospital. We will await her return and hope that she and the baby do well.

6:30pm, only 45 minutes to go. My feet hurt and I am having trouble wrapping up the tasks of the day as my brain is tired as well. As I lift my head, out of the corner of my eye, I see a mostly grey haired woman, wincing in pain in a wheelchair approaching our desk. She is 45 years old and this will be her seventh baby. She is contracting every three minutes.

This is a bit more than a typical day, however, when it rains it pours, and we have to be ready for anything. It's what I love; it's what I hate.

Start to a Different Day

November 11, 2017. 6:50am. My coat is not off, the night charge nurse looks desperate as she hands me three, not one, but three outpatient charts saying that they are all uncomfortable and just walked in over the course of the last 15 minutes. One of them is a few hallways away, as there is no room for her on the overflowing labor wing. Our intern is in the operating room scrubbed in on a cesarean section. The first of the three women was dilated 5 centimeters, her water had not broken and it was her first baby. This should still take some time for her, so on to the next. The next mom is having her fourth baby; her water broke an hour ago. She will likely move fast as she is already 8 centimeters dilated. I call her doctor who is on the way. The last of the three is 7 centimeters. This is just unreal. It is her second baby and she will deliver soon as well.

To my surprise, the first-time mom who was only 5 centimeters delivered first. We had six deliveries before

10:00am that morning and went on to deliver 30 more (not a typo) over the course of the weekend. There is no lack of population growth in Buffalo, NY, for this I am sure. There will always be these types of days. The ones that leave us utterly exhausted and at the same time, in awe.

These crazy days keep your adrenaline pumping. They keep our minds sharp but sometimes beat our bodies up. Being surrounded by an extremely competent staff is what makes this much more comfortable than I know it could be.

"Life and death are one thread, the same line viewed from different sides. "

—Lao Tzu

"Bad things can happen, and often do—but they only take up a few pages of your story; and anyone can survive a few pages."

—James A. Owen

BAD THINGS HAPPEN
CHAPTER 6

I will apologize here for the length of this chapter. These are the sad stories that have left battle scars on my heart. These are the women I will never forget nor do I want to. They have only enriched my experience as a midwife but more importantly as a human being. Remember what I said earlier. These stories are the vast minority, a fraction of a percent of all the births I have witnessed over a career.

Unfortunately, bad things happen in any profession—things beyond our scope of healing, beyond our reach to fix. When you work in a typically "happy-ending" environment, and something goes wrong, it just seems so much worse. Moms and babies are supposed to live, not die. Birth defects, stillbirths, hemorrhages, and difficult deliveries make up a very small percentage of what goes on, but they do happen and the longer you stay within this profession the more you will see.

I love labor and delivery, but sometimes I question why. I have witnessed some heart wrenching events that I would prefer to never repeat and yet I somehow continue to love this profession. Thankfully, the good outweighs the bad—by a landslide. But, in those moments, in that surreal and sad situation, it is hard to see the light.

Many seasoned labor and delivery workers have

witnessed the scenario of the mom who comes in with a ruptured placenta, addicted to drugs, no prenatal care, yet this baby will survive due to the quick actions of the labor and delivery team. We all wonder how this poor baby stands a chance and hope this child can overcome the odds of his or her surroundings. Then, within the same week or month, the opposite woman comes in. She's done everything right in her prenatal care. She takes vitamins, exercises and eats clean as can be. Her baby has no heart rate. How can this be? We see it all the time. It doesn't seem fair and until our dying day we will never understand the reasons behind these scenarios.

One of the saddest, most unspoken issues of what many L&D personnel will come to witness is the sexually abused patient. Sometimes, I almost think it comes as a surprise to the future mother that her body reacts so dramatically. Needless to say, this is not the time or place to address or discuss, but silently our hearts ache for these women. Typically, these women hate pelvic exams. I know none of us enjoy them, but these women have such a hard time. It's much more than physical. Sometimes they go into a childlike state that I suspect must correlate with the age of the abuse. They can not and will not open their legs and if they do, they will typically not keep them open for the exam, but rather shut them on your arm or hand—no matter how gentle you are. They crawl up on the bed in order to escape this intrusion. Their eyes go somewhere else, far away, in order to save them from the pain of the memory of what they may not even be able to recall. Even an epidural does not help with this type of emotional pain. This is so sad and so very complicated.

The following is a short poem, written by a labor and delivery nurse who understands:

LOST SOULS

Hush is the word most often heard
Don't utter a sound when someone's around
Quiet we must be
Our souls never free
The secret's well kept
A little girl wept

—Carol Ator, RN

Please remember as you read this—these are a few out of the thousands of births witnessed. Though these stories are the rare minority, I bet you will somehow relate or know someone who has been impacted by that rare but devastating experience. This is not told to instill fear. This is how it goes sometimes. This is life (and death) and just plain sad.

Boy or Girl?

In my earlier years as a labor and delivery nurse, one of the most heart wrenching deliveries that I remember so vividly resulted in a healthy baby. So what was so heart wrenching? At the moment of birth, one of the first statements is, "It's a girl!" or, "It's a boy!" Even if the sex has been known through ultrasound or other types of testing, this is the moment it becomes real to most parents as they hope the nursery was set up for the correct sex.

This delivery was a bit different. Initially, this baby was pronounced a girl. Everything had gone so well. After a few minutes with mom, the baby was taken to the warmer for a quick check and clean-up. This is the period of time when Vitamin-K injections are given, erythromycin ointment is placed gently into their eyes, and the baby is weighed.

During this particular delivery, the nursery nurse noted that she thinks this baby actually has a penis and is a boy.

Nothing is said aloud in this moment and a call was placed for the neonatal practitioner to come and take a look. Upon further examination, it was determined that this baby had ambiguous genitalia. This means that the baby had both female and male characteristics and would need to have genetic testing to confirm the actual sex. This would take about two weeks. Two weeks!

The news was delivered to the parents. Shock is an understatement. This affected me as much as a stillborn, and although they had a healthy baby, my heart was breaking for them as we could not tell them if their baby was a boy or a girl.

Imagine the phone calls. What do you say to family members, friends, co-workers? "It's a __?__!" Two weeks! That feels like an eternity. Then there is the guilt of having a healthy baby and being upset about how things are playing out. What do they raise their child as? All of the emotions involved in this scenario made it one of the harder ones to digest. Although the baby was healthy and all would be well, my heart hurt for this family more than I expected. This was many years ago and maybe now this scenario would be a bit easier to digest, as gender identity is an active topic with a much greater support network.

Making of an Angel

Amy came to our labor wing for some routine monitoring after she was found to have a breech baby and a borderline low amniotic fluid level. A breech presentation is typically a baby who is not head-down in the pelvis. Most doctors will choose to deliver this baby by cesarean section, especially if it is her first baby. Low fluid can be significant, as the baby has less wiggle room. The cord may inadvertently be compressed and cause decelerations of the baby's heart rate. Low fluid levels are not that uncommon and one of the many reasons a doctor will induce labor.

We were just going to put Amy on the monitor and if the baby looked great, discharge her and bring her back for a C-section in a few days when she would have been a week from her due date.

From a few moments of putting her on the monitor, we on the labor wing knew she would not be going home without delivering her baby. Although the baby was not in an acute state of distress, we knew the baby would not tolerate labor and something was just not right. Breech or not, Amy was going to end up with a C-section.

With her doctor on the way, everything was set for the C-section and we were ready to go. We are fortunate to have neonatal nurse practitioners on staff that are highly skilled and frequently fly to outlying hospitals to pick up sick babies and bring them back to a tertiary care environment for life-saving care. I am always comforted knowing they are on staff. They are the best in their field and if a baby is to be saved, they will do it. I relayed this particular situation to our practitioner and remember saying, "I think this baby will need a bit of help from you," not knowing in that moment the extent of that statement.

Just prior to going back for surgery, Amy's baby had a drop in heart rate which turned the "as soon as possible" C-section into a STAT C-section. Amy would be going under general anesthesia (faster than a spinal) and dad would not be going in with us. In hindsight, a blessing for which I was thankful for as this sad scenario unfolded.

The emergent C-section went very well and baby was out within a few short minutes. Limp and needing what we thought was a few whiffs of oxygen turned into the longest thirty minutes of our lives as Amy's baby would never take a breath of air despite our desperate attempts.

After every possible attempt to ventilate (put air into the lungs) and sustain a heart rate for this 6-pound baby boy, we were unable to resuscitate this baby. After 30 minutes, time of death was noted and the silence of the operating room had everyone feeling as if this were part of a bad dream we hoped we'd all wake up from.

As mom remained sedated under general anesthesia, her dead baby lay just a few feet away. The reality of what just transpired would be even more painful as we now had to tell the young father and first-time grandparents that there was nothing more that could have been done.

The primal cry. Tears flowing uncontrollably. The rest of that day was a blur. Even though it was just a few short months ago as I write this, the memory of what took place remains in a cloud. I'm sure this is a result somewhat similar to what shock does.

The autopsy results finally came. There was some relief in knowing that nothing was going to save this baby. His lungs were coated with a thick, white material similar to vernix. Vernix is a white cheesy coating that protects the baby's skin while inside mom. In this case, the inside of the lungs was coated and there was absolutely no way to ventilate (breathe) for this baby. It became one of the last deliveries that our neonatal nurse practitioner attended. After a long career it was a deal breaker and too difficult to recover from, even though there was nothing more we could have done.

Many people never find out how or why their baby died. This is harder for the family to accept; it makes closure much more difficult.

I hope Amy and her husband have some closure and some hope that future pregnancies will not be affected. This complication is of the rarest. There was only one other documented case to date that we are now aware of.

Side note: Amy did come back and deliver a healthy baby girl about a year and a half later.

Home Birth Gone Wrong

Angela was a sweet girl who had a rough childhood. Dad was an alcoholic and died before he was 40. Angela's mom was a hypochondriac that suffered from mental illness. Munchausen syndrome by proxy is a behavior pattern in which a caregiver (her mother) fabricates, exaggerates, or induces mental or physical health problems in those in their care (Angela). This is a form of child abuse. Angela had been worked up for every illness imaginable as her mother was sure she had them.

Nothing was ever found, but Angela probably had more invasive medical procedures than most of us will have in a lifetime.

Maybe her history was part of the reason Angela had a fear of hospitals. Angela struggled with obesity and the complications and inconvenience of weighing more than 400 pounds for her 5'4" height.

Angela met a nice man and although they never married, Jeff was supportive and hardworking.

When Angela became pregnant with her first child, she would have panic attacks about the thoughts of once again being in the hospital. She postponed her prenatal care to avoid this dilemma. She had lots of time, right?

Weeks turned into months, months turned into a full term pregnancy, and due to Angela's size, most of her friends and co-workers did not even know she was pregnant.

Angela had done some research and reading. Childbirth was a natural process that typically resulted in a bit of labor and then a baby. Women all through history were having babies in their home, why couldn't she?

Angela had decided that she was going to have a home birth. Jeff was a bit reluctant but felt it was ultimately her decision. Besides, one of their neighbors was a nurse if they needed help.

It all started as a backache and reminded her of period cramps from oh so long ago. Eventually the contractions began and for the first eight hours, Angela thought she could definitely do this.

After a day and a half, Angela could take no more and it wasn't hard for Jeff to talk her into a trip to the hospital. At the registration desk Jeff reported that they had no doctor and Angela had been in labor for almost two days.

I know what is going through the staff's mind right now. Is she crazy? Is she even pregnant? Is she pre-term? Where do we even begin? For us, it is starting from scratch which is hard to do when you have someone presenting this uncomfortable. We know nothing about her.

Angela was taken to the exam room. A few minutes later the nurse called out for the sonogram machine as she could not find a heartbeat. Due to Angela's size, this is not an abnormal finding and we still have no proof that she is even pregnant. It has happened, more than you would think, that we have received "labor" patients who are not even pregnant.

The resident began the ultrasound. Yes, there was a baby. It looked to be a good size. The room got quiet when the baby's heart was located and there was no activity, no heart beat. When did this baby die? We will never know for sure, but may have an idea when the baby is delivered and we see the condition of the skin.

Everyone hates this scenario. Angela is in shock and Jeff cries silently. The staff is so quick to judge and become angry; this did not have to happen. But they have not walked in Angela's shoes. This is something Angela will now have to live with and work through.

The nurse was upset, as Angela was fully dilated and would not push. She was most likely in shock and needed time. The baby would eventually come. This is such a sad, sad scenario.

One Baby, No Mother

I cannot remember her name as it was more than 20 years ago, but I remember that she was 17-years-old and single. Her boyfriend slept soundly in the chair beside her, not disturbed by what was going on around him.

In early labor, her doctor decided to break her water. This is a common procedure to facilitate a more rapid labor. It has its pros and cons, but would definitely not be described as dangerous or uncommon. As long as the baby's head is well applied to the cervix and is low enough in the pelvis, this usually works out well.

As is the norm, we put her in a flat position and have her open her legs for a pelvic exam. Breaking the water (amniotomy) is not a painful procedure. It is done with a tool that looks like a long crochet hook, which looks much worse than anything it could to. It takes about 3 seconds, typically.

On this day, one that we would never forget, her water was broken and within minutes she at straight up and stated she could not breathe. The situation became emergent and desperate in seconds. This poor girl went from respiratory arrest into cardiac arrest in a very short amount of time. As she was wheeled back to the operating room for an emergency cesarean section, a nurse rode the cart with her, doing chest compressions all the way.

Within minutes, a baby boy was born, needing some resuscitation but eventually took a breath and cried. Something his mother, lying only a few feet away, would never do again.

Amniotic fluid embolism is a rare obstetric emergency in which amniotic fluid, fetal cells, hair, or other debris enters the mother's bloodstream via the placental bed of the uterus and trigger an allergic reaction. This reaction then results in cardiorespiratory collapse and coagulopathy. Coagulopathy, in this case, referred to a bleeding condition that could not be kept up with

After an hour of attempts, this mother lost her battle to a rare but lethal condition that almost every seasoned labor and delivery nurse hopes to never see, or ever see again.

A baby without a mother.

Megan's Story

On July 12th, 2010 I arrived early in the morning as scheduled to begin my shift as a midwife. Little did I know the events that would take place that day would affect many of us like never before. The day started with a full labor wing, nowhere to put arrivals, and you just do your best to provide all that you can.

There was a couple in Birthing Room 2 that I had not yet met face to face, but was informed that her bloodwork had come back with very abnormal results. I went in to meet this girl who proceeded to tell me that she felt fine, besides being a little tired, as many women at nine months are. The blood count did not match the picture of the beautiful, vibrant healthy girl in early labor that I had in front of me. Lab error?

Must be. We repeated the lab work and unfortunately got the same results. Just two weeks prior, Megan had normal bloodwork.

Her doctor and a hematologist were notified and before Megan was halfway through her labor, a well known local cancer institute, Roswell Park Comprehensive Cancer Center, was holding a bed for her on their leukemia unit. Megan was to be transferred immediately following delivery.

Shocked was an understatement. The rest of the day was a blur. Her husband sat helpless as the day unraveled and filled us with mixed emotions. Plans were made to collect the cord blood as it may come in handy sometime in the near future. Approximately 10:00pm that evening after 3 long hours of pushing, a beautiful 7 pound, 3 ounce baby girl came into the world. Within hours, Megan was transferred to Roswell. This is where her battle with AML (acute myeloid leukemia) was about to begin. Two days after her birth, I went to see this amazing girl. On oxygen as she was suffering from a noninfectious pneumonia, she was grateful and felt so optimistic that this was found so early. I was infinitely touched by her beauty, strength and optimism.

Two days later, she was placed in a drug induced coma, placed on a ventilator (breathing machine) in order to begin aggressive chemotherapy. Things like this just don't happen on the labor wing.

Approximately 3 months later, Megan lost her battle to this aggressive and rare form of cancer. Within all of the sadness there formed a circle of human beings with incredible strength and faith. I am in awe and was honored to know these people. Thanks to social media, I am able to see Megan's little girl grow up to be as beautiful as her mother.

Not So Merry Christmas
Jessica was expecting her first baby. I recall that her due date fell on Christmas day. It was a girl. Jessica's doctor called us from his office and told us he was sending in a patient, days before her due date, with no fetal heart rate.

Your first reaction is to run for the hills. I don't want this patient. This is too sad and it's Christmas! This selfish, self-centered feeling leaves quickly as you come face to face with a mother who just had her heart ripped out. Sometimes the sadness is so raw, you cannot speak. You just hold on. You are just there, a support, something real among the shock.

Jessica was induced and delivered the next day. The baby girl was beautiful, as they usually are. Born without an obvious reason why or how this could have happened. This is so hard when there are no answers.

These are the patients you never ever forget. Maybe it is the pure strength of getting through something like this that leaves the rest of us awestruck.

Later that year, Jessica was again pregnant. It's hard to imagine what goes through their minds. How do they not worry about every little thing? Toward the end of Jessica's pregnancy, she would have frequent ultrasounds so we were able to connect on a regular basis.

Holidays seemed to hold a theme for Jessica as I believe she went in on Valentine's Day to deliver a healthy baby boy and since then, another baby girl.

Any seasoned labor nurse will tell you that it is not uncommon to see the family who experienced the devastating loss of a baby have a baby about a year after their loss. This is not something I recommend mentioning at the time of the loss, as grief contains no room for this possibility. At the very least, it is a reminder that life does go on even after it appears to stand still, stuck in sadness.

Too Early To Lose

Occasionally on the labor wing, we have the sad job of inducing a woman when a fetal death has occurred mid-pregnancy. Another scenario is that we have a baby who has anomalies (defects) that will not likely survive the pregnancy or live long after birth. This scenario is brought up in front of an ethics committee for approval, as we are inducing labor in a baby that still has a heartbeat. This is where your beliefs and judgement have to stay at home. It is not ours to judge and we are not walking in this woman's shoes.

After a slow and gentle admission, we begin the induction by using something such as Cytotec which is in capsule form for oral and vaginal use. It can be repeated every four hours until delivery is achieved.

What seems so unfair to me is that this process can take days. Why does this mom not only have to go through the loss of her baby, but the duration of the process as well? Again, I have no answers. We offer the mom anything she wants for pain but what typically happens does not allow time for an epidural.

Once the mom becomes uncomfortable, things usually happen fast. This is why her doctor won't likely be there for the delivery and why the midwife or resident usually will. Remember, you do not need to be fully dilated to deliver a baby that weighs less than a pound.

For all of our admissions of fetal loss, the discussion of holding the baby comes up. Initially, this conversation horrifies the family, then becomes the most important part of closure and grieving.

I have noticed over the years that many couples fear seeing the baby as it will not resemble a human or a deformity will be traumatic to look at. The opposite is actually true. What people imagine is often much more exaggerated than what actually is. Most parents find such comfort in holding their little one, even for such a short moment in time.

Most L&D personnel have been trained to help you through this very delicate time and most often, deep emotional bonds and connections are made that do not seem to happen under normal circumstances. As a labor and delivery nurse, the typical thought is, I don't want that patient. This has nothing to do with the patient at all. This is a response to the emotions that we know we have to face up to, which are not always comfortable. This initial discomfort often evolves into, "I love this patient and I will never forget them."

Life Comes Full Circle

Keri is a 40-year-old Hospice nurse. She worked hard for this pregnancy, as she thought she was finished reproducing 19 years ago. Who could ask for more—a girl and a boy, two years apart and life was good. That is, until last year when their 20-year-old daughter was taken from them in a tragic car accident.

I write this piece, in the most difficult chapter, almost in the moment. This is one of those deliveries you feel that it was a gift to be at. I want to send the family a thank you note for allowing me the opportunity to be present at this birth. Beautiful is an understatement when describing this birth. It was raw and powerful. It was miraculous and it was healing. It was absolutely one of the most touching births I have been privileged to hold to memory. A piece of Heaven was surely in the room.

Keri's 19-year-old son, surely traumatized by the loss of his older sister, sits quietly. What could be going through that head of his? A horrific loss and a new life about to come full circle. I had no idea what to expect from him. He would leave the room every time his mom was examined out of politeness and a calm maturity that is uncommon for his age. He and his dad seemed to have quite a bond, as I'm sure they all did. They had lived through something none of us can even imagine. They were solid, this was palpable.

One of the most memorable and powerful moments in all of this was when Keri was checked and found to be fully dilated. Everything felt right. The head was low, and I felt she would barely push for 10 minutes. She was comfortable with her epidural and so grateful for it. I looked up at this beautiful mom-to-be and asked, "Are you ready?" Her face flushed and tears welled from her eyes. Emotions that are so hard to describe flooded that room in that moment—the pain of the most tremendous loss and the joy of what is only a few minutes away. My heart ached and my eyes couldn't help but fill right along with hers.

That wonderful dad and dedicated husband became a bit faint during the delivery. I vividly remember the grey and paste-like color of his skin. He immediately sat down and probably has trouble recalling what happened next. Can you even imagine the emotion of it all? A big brother, in awe of it all, steps up to cut the cord and watch as his beautiful sister makes her way into their lives.

Beautiful and comedic distractions made for not only a memorable delivery, but a moment in time that no one in the room will ever forget. For this sweet family who has been bound by life's greatest tragedy finally shared one of life's most beautiful miracles.

Perfect Labor, Perfect Delivery, Not So Perfect Outcome

Laura and Jim were first-time parents who were anxiously awaiting the arrival of their little (or not so little) baby girl. Laura's labor was progressing very well and that little baby girl could not have looked more perfect on the monitor. She had not even the slightest dip of heart rate while pushing. This was the couple that you loved to be with. Dad was a bit skittish but once we started pushing, he stepped right up to the plate and was actually a great coach. The energy and atmosphere in this room is what makes me love this job. After only 20 minutes of pushing, I had to get her doctor in as she was doing so well and it wouldn't be long. After pushing a short 45 minutes, Laura delivered a beautiful baby girl 15 minutes before my shift ended. It was a perfect send off for the start of my vacation. I love my job!

The next morning, I received a text from Laura's doctor saying Laura's baby was transferred to Children's Hospital with a massive brain bleed. I was stunned as this was the most beautiful delivery. What happened? She did not push long and there were no complications. As I write this piece, a few weeks later, the baby is still not doing well. The consensus so far is a congenital malformation within the brain. I pray for these sweet parents.

Life is really not fair sometimes. Life emerges and life ends. Either way, we go on, having very little control of the outcome or timing. It is a gift to experience moments such as these. Even the bad outcomes move you in a beautiful and indescribable way and reinforce how precious life is.

I dedicate this chapter to all women who have known loss such as this. I'm not sure where your strength comes from or even how you breathe. There are no words.

"I've learned that when you try to control everything, you enjoy nothing."

—Unknown

"You can't control everything. Sometimes you just need to relax and have faith that things will work out. Let go a little and just let life happen."

—Unknown

"As long as everything is the way I want it, I'm totally flexible."

—Unknown

THE BIRTH PLAN
CHAPTER 7

This is such a hot topic in the land of labor and delivery. The birth plan, originally designed to help coordinate a mother and father's birth choices and desires, has spun so far out of control that most labor nurses cringe when they hear the word.

If you are familiar with the HGTV show "Love It or List It" then you may be able to relate to my interpretation of the birth plan. I'm neither for or against the birth plan, however, the more specific or detailed the list is, the harder it becomes to accommodate everything on your list. I feel that as your labor and delivery staff, we go into the process optimistic and all-in to provide you with the experience you desire. Then, along the way, we will have to cross things off your list in order to keep going in the right direction.

Most birth plans are realistic and not far off the mark for what we do on a daily basis anyway. Low lighting, music, prefers no pain medications, who will be in the room, and so on. Many prefer to not cut the umbilical cord until it stops pulsating, this is reasonable and most of us are happy to oblige. Many hospitals are now eliminating the "nursery" and keeping babies with you at all times.

First, can we define "natural?" I'd bet money that all of our definitions of a natural childbirth are significantly different. Mine would probably be on the more lenient side. I would define a natural childbirth as "any birth via the vaginal route unassisted by forceps or a vacuum." Having an epidural or the use of Pitocin to augment things does not disqualify you from having natural birth in my eyes, in my opinion. It is still the most beautiful moment in time. Many of you will not agree, but walk in my shoes for as many years as I have, and you will appreciate birth in its many varieties. It is the people in the room that make it a beautiful experience, or not, no matter the details.

The following birth plan examples can be used as a great reference while writing your own. Remember, when you start to get too specific on how you want things to go, you set yourself up for failure which is not fair to you or those taking care of you.

There are many online resources to guide you when it comes to writing a birth plan if you chose to do so. My advice is to go over this with your provider(s) prior to your admission to the hospital. This may allow some alternate perspective for you to consider and puts you on a level playing field. Many physicians are blindsided by some of their patients requests as it was never discussed prior to delivery.

Birth Plan: Go Team!

The following is one of the more unrealistic birth plans that put our staff on the defense before we even meet the patient. This is probably one of the most extreme plans I have ever seen and I'm so grateful to not be a part of. I am angry before I even meet her. Not many nurses would sign up for this patient. I will comment after each request as to what the majority of labor and delivery personnel would be thinking as they read this:

Thank you for being a part of my birth team! Below are a few items I'd like you to keep in mind and help me out with during my labor. Let's make a romantic and memorable event in my life and yours! It's going to be a fairy tale come true. —I think the author of this birth plan is trying to get her "team" on the same page. So far not too bad…

I wish to be photographed and videotaped throughout the entire process, although not continuously. Please remind me to fix my hair and clothes. _____ will be my fashion manager. —What? Most of us don't mind helping to capture some great photos, but really, a fashion manager? Good thing you have one as it will take the pressure off of us. And this is your #1?

____ and ____ will need to take food breaks and rest at regular intervals. —Good for them, we don't need to know this. Bring food for them or follow the signs to the cafeteria.

I want roses. I want music playing continuously. —I hope you remember to bring them in.

I will try to sleep through as much early labor as I can. —No problem because according to you, you will not be coming in until you are very active.

I will not utilize breathing techniques until the rising intensity demands them. —Okay.

I prefer to use more primal and emotional expressions such as crying and talking to baby through much of my labor. —Okay, but please try not to swear or scare the other patients.

I will have enemas at some point before coming to the hospital. —Fine by us, but sometimes that can backfire.

I do not wish to go to the hospital until at least 5cm dilated. —How do you plan on knowing this? Maybe your photographer can check you. None of my staff makes house calls. Most women having their first baby are pretty uncomfortable by the time they are 4 centimeters. Our advice is to stay home as long as possible so you can put your birth plan into action there.

Food DO's: Try to make everything at or above room temperature unless I absolutely have to have something cold to calm down a burning uterus. Wine, rice wine, food pre-cooked by myself, fresh coconut, fruits, and veggies, warm soup, herbal tea, skim milk and birds nest, breakfast cereal.
—We'd like to know how long you are planning on being in labor. Since you are coming in after you are 5 centimeters, your stomach will not digest all of this. It's OK, we are happy to give your birth partner and fashion manager buckets to hold while you puke your brains out while crying and talking to your baby. I am all for eating in early labor, but once things get busy, eating does not usually go well.

Food DON'Ts: Try to avoid plain water, ice chips or anything below room temperature. —Most moms love ice chips in transitional labor. We hope you plan on bringing in your own non-plain water as we only tend to have the plain version.

If it is a warm day, I'd like some outdoor time and outdoor pictures. — Our recommendation would be to shoot those pictures before you step into the hospital. We are usually caring for more than one person and won't be able to assist you and your posse outside. We're not thinking you will be much in the mood for outside pictures past 5 centimeters.

I wish to be touched as little as possible by the medical staff. I want the least amount of vaginal exams. —Okay, but most women respond very well, and as a matter of fact, never forget the touch of their labor nurse. We are very curious at this point as to why you are not having a home birth.

I DO NOT want to hear anything about pain medication. If I have a meltdown from the pain, I'd like to be told to "snap out of it." — Seriously? We could be written up for that.

I wish to have the attending doctor deliver my baby instead of the intern.

—No problem.

Lots of pictures of my baby at my bosom but avoid nipple shots, be creative. —We are pretty sure your fashion manager will take care of this. We are not photographers.

I want to have a good look at the placenta before it is sent to the lab. — Sure, no problem. We are just glad you don't want to eat it!

My Baby is not to leave my or my partner's sight. My paranoia is immense because I have put an enormous effort into cultivating this fine product. — Poor thing and poor baby. We are sure you are the only woman in history to work so hard in cultivating your fine "product." It is so hard to read this without nausea.

Have Fun! Go Team! —This is no team we want to be a part of. You are most likely very self centered and care very little for anyone around you. We are sad for your baby, a human being, not a product or a doll to pose with. Of course we will take care of you but you will make us question our job and our love of our job.

Follow Up
The nurse caring for this patient actually had to turn her over to another as she was extremely rude. This is not surprising considering the tone of this birth plan.

Even a year after I initially wrote this piece, I am sad at the tone of this, including my response as you can palpate my disgust which is not typical for me. I am usually not a cynical person, yet this birth plan brought out the worst in me. I wonder how her "fine product" is doing.

Not Our Typical Birth Plan
This birth plan was written by a 21-year-old girl. Moms this young do not typically write birth plans as they are more go-with-the-flow:

I would like an epidural as soon as possible. —Funny thing was, as soon as she asked for her epidural, a code blue was called. The anesthesiologist was called away to save a life. No worries as she did eventually get her epidural. We actually don't have a problem with this request.

If labor slows down, I would like medication to speed it up. —This is a first for us. Most moms prefer to avoid Pitocin.

I DO NOT want an episiotomy if at all possible. —Okay, we will try as fewer and fewer are being done and it's not standard of care. Episiotomies are actually frowned upon these days.

I'd like the lights in the delivery room to be dim and quiet. —We don't have noise lights. This request is fine.

If I have to have a C-Section, I'd like to be put under and be the first person to hold the baby please. No one else. —I hope she is referring to her family and not the staff. Are we supposed to leave the baby on the table until she wakes up? Waking up from general anesthesia is much more uncomfortable than if you have a spinal and there is less risk for the baby.

I'd like the doctor to cut the cord. —Unusual, but we understand.

I do not want to breastfeed. —That is your decision.

I actually applaud the honesty of this young mom. She probably is more afraid than a control freak. Just some kind education could soften this up a bit. She will do and be fine.

Our Fun Resident
Bianca was one of our favorite residents. Her sense of humor always brightened our day. When it came for her to start her own beautiful family, she came in, birth plan in hand, and ready to go:

Environment:
We would like mood lighting.

The following people who were with us at conception, will be with us today; Marcus, Bianca's mom, Marcus' mom, a couple of Bianca's friends and Anthony Muney (a fellow resident).

In lieu of a traditional hospital gown, we both prefer to be naked...on admission.

Prep:
Bianca would prefer no shaving or enema. If shaving is necessary, we prefer something in the shape of a money sign. Marcus' pubic hair should not be shaved.

Marcus will need an IV.

Bianca would like an epidural when she is closed, thick and high, in the car, on Maple Rd. (Hospital is on Maple Rd).

She would also like an episiotomy upon registration at nurses' station. In triage, only Anthony Muney will be allowed to examine my cervix.

We prefer the labor bed to be a Sleep Number bed.

Labor:
Bianca would like Marcus to do the pushing whenever possible. We will both be doing Lamaze breathing.

No amniotomy (artificial rupture of membranes) is to be performed, my baby will perform amniotomy when he is ready.

We do not want doctors, residents, nurses, midwives or doulas present, only medical students please.

We chose doctor Metchler because he shares our philosophy in a natural, low intervention birth. Dr. Metchler will deliver the baby via skype from his home theater.

If Marcus starts to sob uncontrollably, please turn off "The Notebook". If he continues to cry please administer the following drugs per Dr. Metchler: Demerol, Ativan, Nubian, and medical marijuana.

We would like gangster rap to be played throughout the labor process except when baby is crowning we will switch to classical music.

Fetal electronic monitoring only if it's a Tuesday.

Breast feeding to start at +2 station (as baby's head is almost crowning).

Delivery:
We strongly prefer a boy.

Only break the bed after the baby's arms are delivered.

After placenta is delivered naturally, no cutting or pulling. Baby will remain attached to placenta until 1st birthday.

I would like my baby, myself, Marcus, Dr. Mechtler, labor nurses, and nursery nurses to all receive Vitamin-K shots and erythromycin ointment.

Post birth:
Marcus is to skin-to-skin immediately after baby is born.

Please do not weigh our baby, as we do not want our baby to have the same body issues as her fat mom.

We ask that the baby is bathed in our presence, in our delivery room, in Perrier.

I love her sense of humor. She was always lovely to be around. So wherever you are Dr. Bianca, we miss you.

I Will, I Want, I Expect

I want you to read the following birth plan. I will keep my mouth shut (so hard) as you read, but I want you to see how it makes you feel. Do you want to be around this person? Do you feel the love, or are you repelled? For moms-to-be who are considering a birth plan, see how this makes you feel. Remember, we sometimes meet your birth plan before we meet you. I'm sure that some of this is lost in translation. But the gist of this birth plan is not positive or welcoming. It leaves the staff dreading the day she walks through the door:

During my labor I do not want to be cared for by: Resident Medical Students, Graduate Nurses who have not yet received license, LPN's, Midwives in training who have not yet received certification, and will refuse any medical or nursing care provided by males with the possible exception of an anesthesiologist.

I would prefer to receive care by Certified Nurse Midwives rather than RN's who are not yet Certified Nurse Midwives.

I would like to receive as few cervical assessments as possible during my labor.

During my labor I would prefer to have a saline lock in place, however I plan on drinking my liquids rather than receiving IV hydration and fluid boluses, I am aware that Pitocin may become part of the induction process and have received IV Pitocin without receiving IV fluids previously at (another hospital).

I want intermittent fetal monitoring during my labor so that I can move about with liberty to change positions to facilitate fetal positioning for birth.

I will refuse AROM (artificial rupture of membranes) before active labor has commenced and prefer not to be offered AROM.

I will request pain medication and do not want to be offered or encouraged to receive pain medications before I request them. I have accepted Nubain in previous labors and may request an epidural at 7 centimeters dilation. If I do request an epidural, I would like it turned off so that I may feel the urge to push. I may request a pudendal block before pushing and delivery even though I would like to avoid episiotomy. —I can't hold back here. I have not seen a doctor perform a pudendal block in over 20+ years. If you want to be a guinea pig for something that I'm sure your doctor has not done, have at it!

I expect to be allowed to shower during labor as a non-pharmacological pain intervention.

I would like my husband to be present at liberty throughout induction and labor and any discussions involving my and the healthcare of our unborn baby. All discussions should be directed to us as a couple and not to either as a single party.

I only want the minimum amount of staff present in the room at the time of birth, and I do not want students of any variety observing any part of induction, labor, delivery and postpartum. —Read below for why she needed to have more people at delivery.

I do not want coached pushing; I prefer to push when I feel the urge to do so.

I do not want to push in stirrups and do not want anyone holding my legs while I am pushing.

I may prefer to push and deliver with my own arms wrapped around my knees.

I may ask for peanut style yoga/birthing ball near the end of labor.

Our baby will breastfeed and I do not want him to receive supplemental nutrition following birth. I have successfully exclusively breastfed my 2 other children and would not like to be bothered by frequent interruptions from a lactation consultant. If I have any problems or questions about nursing my baby, then I will request a lactation consultant at that point.

I would like to nurse my baby immediately following birth and have skin to skin contact at that time.

I would like my baby to stay in the room with me postpartum rather than being kept in the nursery.

We would like our child to be circumcised.

So, what did you think? Do you want to care for this person? Demanding and rude is the undertone, and I, as the ONLY Certified Nurse Midwife on staff (on a busy day) wanted nothing to do with her. Most of her requests were reasonable but the undertone was not. A great teaching patient for the intern.

Oh, and by the way, because she was essentially a non-compliant patient who basically ignored her gestational diabetic condition, she grew a 10lb baby that had something called shoulder dystocia at delivery. Shoulder dystocia is potentially a very serious and sometimes deadly situation in which the head delivers, but we cannot deliver the big shoulders in a timely manner. This is an "all hands on deck" situation where everyone available is in the room to help the delivering doctor get this baby out. So we will push your knees back to your ears, flip you over and do anything else it takes to help get your baby out alive. And we did. We are sorry that we went against your plan for minimal staff in the room, and your wishes to immediately breastfeed were not followed in order to resuscitate your baby. Aside from some postpartum blood sugar issues, this jumbo baby did well. So did mom.

Summary

My best advice for the parents-to-be is to look at the birth plan as your wish list. Remember, our goals are the same: healthy mom, healthy baby. The tighter the controls and more specific your details are, the more likely you are setting yourself up for disappointment. This leaves everyone feeling bad. The staff in charge of your care as well as your doctor have very little control over how your labor will play out, but it is their experience and expertise that will get you through it. The patients that seem to have the best labor and delivery experience are the ones that come in with more of a go-with-the-flow attitude.

One of the funniest plans I have seen was short and sweet, "Two people come in to have a baby. Three people leave. No one dies." I did laugh out loud, but I think I prefer a gentler version, "Two people come in to have a baby. Three people leave happy and healthy."

"Crazy things happen when there is a full moon."
                                        —Everyone in Healthcare

PUSH

STORMS, FULL MOONS & WACKY WEATHER
CHAPTER 8

Weather definitely has an impact on our body and mood. Most fail to realize how "in-tune" to weather that they actually are. It doesn't take a meteorologist to tell you that your joints ache or your sinuses are acting up.

Thanks to gravity, we have fairly constant pressure applied to our body at all times—14.6 pounds of pressure per square inch (at sea level) to be exact. When the barometric pressure drops, your support has loosened up, per se. It's like wearing a knee brace, then losing some support when it comes off.

With bad weather, there is usually a drop in barometric pressure. This is extreme in situations such as a hurricanes or snowstorms. People who are chronically inflamed will feel changes in the weather before anyone else.

Low barometric pressure that results from an impending storm does seem to affect the onset of natural labor, as well rupture of membranes. As with the full moon, the studies do not support this as much as health care providers would swear by.

As I write this particular piece (November 2014),

Buffalo, NY is under a state of emergency four days after a record breaking snowfall paralyzed so many people in its southern suburbs. I thankfully live 30 miles north of this "Snowvember" disaster. 85 inches seems to be the final tally. Even for Buffalo, this is more of a winter average, not an event average. Many people were stuck on the thruway for more than 36 hours while their cars were buried under 5-7 feet of snow. In my 30+ years of living in Western New York, I have never seen the I-90/I-190 (local thruway) closed for more than three days. This was incredible!

As I recall, I posted to Facebook a prediction that came to be just two days prior to the event. There was a prediction for a snow event in Western New York. Many times, the local meteorologists tend to over forecast a weather event or at least during the past year, predict amazingly wrong. My gut knew they were on to something this time. It was a Sunday, my weekend on at the hospital. I am the only midwife on without an intern. Thankfully, I am surrounded by a very competent nursing staff that usually makes the unbearable manageable. The in-house attendant is there, but is of no help when it comes to assessing, admitting and managing patients. However, in the event of an emergency, I am very thankful that their body is in the building. But for the sake of being busy, I feel very alone and overwhelmed on this particular day.

My shifts typically start at 6:45am. On this particular Sunday, I had already admitted four patients and it wasn't even 8:00am. Oh my gosh, this was going to be a long day. To top it off, I was already in a bad mood (rare for me) as one of my new patients did not speak English and her husband did not feel like helping interpret for me. As I tried to admit her, he wanted to leave. I sternly informed him that he would not be leaving until I had the information I needed. Once I had all I needed I told him he was free to go, silently (and maybe obviously) disgusted that he would leave his wife in such a vulnerable position. Yes, we do have interpreter phones, but his desire to bolt was just mind boggling as his wife was just plain scared-to-death. You may be thinking, it might just be a cultural thing, but you were not there to feel the vibe I was getting. I did not like him.

The day went on and by 5:00pm I had admitted my 12th labor patient. When things like this happen, there is typically a full moon in our near future, a storm brewing, or a surge that is taking place nine months after an unusual weather event. Not that I had time to watch the news, but on this day, an unusually early snow event was being anticipated and said to begin within the next 24-48 hours. It was not even Thanksgiving yet and certainly not winter. Even Buffalonians are not prepared for an event such as this. 1-2 feet of snow were being predicted and my gut said they were going to be right. Unfortunately, the predicted snowfall totals were actually 4-5 feet less than what actually fell in some areas. Many lives were lost, roofs collapsed, schools and businesses closed, all of which affected so many people. The National Guard was even brought in to help.

Health Care Personnel are usually the exclusion when it comes to a driving ban. No snow days for us. Under the circumstance of that infamous November storm, many were unable to show up as it was physically impossible to walk out of their doors. Buffalo is a very unique place. When life gets difficult, you want to know someone from Buffalo. These people show their true colors when the going gets tough

Buffalo people in general are built strong and kind. Many people who leave the area for warmer climates have eventually come back as they miss the kind of people that makes this part of the state so great.

This is only one of many weather related, barometric pressure dropping, water breaking, labor inducing events that any labor and delivery team player sees on a regular basis.

As I write this book, I attempt to research actual data that supports what I say. There is very little. So for all of you "left brain" individuals that need the concrete, black and white evidence; just come and see it for yourselves. There is no seasoned labor and delivery nurse that would dispute this, or any medical personnel as well.

Moon Drama

It has been my experience that it is not the actual full moon that increases the nursery volume by 10's and 20's, but more so in the few days prior to the full moon.

Contrary to what most believe, including myself, there has been no valid scientific study to support the effect of the moon when it comes to birth or even life on Earth. I bet that animals would even disagree. For anyone who has ever been employed within the walls of a hospital, saying the moon does not play a role on volume or wackiness is like saying there is no God and unlike God, we can see the moon.

In my world, the cycle of the moon correlates with the menstrual cycle which averages 28 days. Coincidence?

I have read at least 20 studies on this and am actually stunned that there was not strong evidence to support lunar effect on birth, medical conditions, and even behavior. I don't think I am alone, but it is possible that we notice more during the full moon and tend to disregard the abnormal when there is not a moon to blame.

Let it Rain

When there is significant rainfall predicted in the near future, expect those uteri to give way as well. Premature rupture of membranes is a frequent occurrence with torrential rains. Premature rupture of membranes refers to the "breaking of the water" and labor does not follow as it typically would. Pitocin or some other form of induction usually entails.

Even a Solar Eclipse

I was lucky to find myself scheduled on August 21st, 2017 for the solar eclipse. Although Buffalo was not in the 100% eclipse zone, it was enough to cause a ruckus on our labor wing especially in the form of preterm labor and women in labor who had a previous cesarean section. When I polled a labor and delivery online group, the consensus for the most part was the same.

If I am fortunate enough to still be working and loving my job in 2024, I will avoid April 8 as that is the scheduled date of the next solar eclipse. I will let the younger, more energetic co-workers enjoy all the activity.

I LOVE WEATHER! Next to labor and delivery I find weather events fascinating. Maybe a career in meteorology is in store for me in my next life.

"When you're a nurse you know that every day you will touch a life or a life will touch yours."

—Unknown

"They may forget your name, but they will NEVER FORGET how you made them feel."

—Maya Angelou

ANATOMY OF A LABOR NURSE
CHAPTER 9

It is no secret that in order to get a position on the Labor and Delivery Unit, someone has to retire (or die) as this area of nursing has an incredible disposition for longevity. This makes seasoned labor nurses, at times, far more experienced and knowledgeable than your doctor when it comes to the ins and outs of labor. In the teaching institutions, July comes around and the new interns show up. Some scared to death, some cocky, some competent, and some should never be there in the first place. It is in the new interns' best interest, and learning potential, to treat these seasoned nurses like their mother, sister or best friend. This will go a long way in buffering this long and painful year. The "seasoned nurse" will take good care of them if they don't piss her off at hello. If they do, I am not responsible for how rough things can get. Be wary new intern, you may not know who is responsible for your evaluation. She may even protect you from the more difficult attending physicians if she likes you.

I apologize if I offend any male labor and delivery nurses by always using the pronoun "she." I did know and was trained by a male midwife, but in all my years, I have never worked with a male labor nurse.

For the most part (with some exceptions, of course) labor nurses need the least advice when it comes to keeping you safe. They have most likely been doing this longer than your doctor and I'll bet large sums of money that their mediation has saved many patients from unnecessary surgery or intervention. And they do it so well, the physician did not even realize the nurse intervened on your behalf.

I am NOT disregarding or devaluing the necessity of our doctors as they are the ones who will save the day when the going gets tough. When it comes to hands on experience, the nurse plays a huge role in how this labor will go down. Most OB/GYNs are not in the room until, as they say, "don't call me 'til you see the eyebrows." Of course I'm exaggerating a bit, but the attending OB doctor just does not have the time to sit with the patient through labor or possibly two hours of pushing. If they did, patients would have never met them in the office. It is that precious nurse that protects, supports and cheers you on for hours and sometimes even days.

The L&D nurse is built tough. No wusses allowed and they live for adrenaline rushes whether they admit it or not. Forget being squeamish, there is no room for this as a labor and delivery nurse. Most of them have a great sense of humor that some may consider morbid. Things get crazy!

To qualify for this position, you need to exhibit the ultimate multitasking skill set, eat in motion, and have a bladder capacity that defies the biggest balloon you can imagine. The labor and delivery nurse can muster up super human strength in order to turn women three times her size, with an epidural, in a single maneuver. Husbands will watch in awe.

They will have hands in places you have never imagined, get splattered with all kinds of human debris, and still manage not to bat an eye. They are peed on, pooped on, and will take many showers in eau-de-amniotic fluid. By tomorrow, they forget, and even if they bump into said patient in the supermarket—they don't remember the uncomfortable details that tend to stick with patient, we promise.

Labor nurses develop super human senses and can hear a drop in a baby's heart rate from the other site of the unit. This is an amazing gift that evolves over time and was in place long before central fetal monitoring took over.

Labor nurses rarely eat in the cafeteria. They eat when they can, sometimes even standing. They can talk about blood clots and placentas as they take a famished bite of whatever may be in the fridge and it may have been there a good long time. She is hungry and desperate; she'll eat anything (except maybe your placenta). They frequently suffer from constipation and urinary tract infections as they remain loyal to you over their own bodily functions.

Anyone who has been working labor and delivery for a bit will relate, and even recognize themselves when we stereotype the labor nurse. Much gratitude goes to the thousands of members of the Facebook group, "Labor & Delivery Nurses Rock" for their fast and fun contributions. The descriptions below became a collective experience that anyone working in this area will relate to. They made my job here much easier and helped fuel the inspiration behind this book. This we know; we can work in any labor wing in North America (and probably the world) and still find the stereotypes listed below.

So now, for your nursing cast of characters, I present you with (in no particular order):

The Procrastinator: The nurse that appears to do everything within her power to prevent the patient from delivering on her shift. This nurse will usually come in early and choose the patient on the board that is least likely to deliver.

The Pain Monitor: This nurse seems to know how much pain you are in. We're not sure how she does it, but she will tell you when you are in pain or real labor regardless of how you feel. This irritates me to no end. It is the patient's perception that we care about, so even if you think you are in the worst pain ever and we know things will get worse, we should treat and manage your perception, not ours.

The Meconium (Shit) Magnet: There is a charge nurse I will call LOLA. Every unit has one. Lola is probably one of the best nurses I know, but when she is not in charge and actually has a patient, we will be watching closely. She can administer the most difficult IV—blindfolded. Lola has a knack for attracting the patient that will most likely become the STAT patient or some other adrenaline-producing scenario. Her patients always love her, as do we, but you cannot help noticing that she is the common denominator when meconium (shit) happens. When she is in charge, the unit is typically at or above capacity.

The Ultimate Documenter: This nurse is so focused on documentation, we swear she could miss the delivery and not know it. This type of nurse typically has a fear of doing something wrong. Maybe she has deep feeling of not being good enough so she always has to double check. Obstetrics is one area of health care that has a high litigation rate. Maybe fear of litigation is a motivator, but this nurse takes things to a new level.

The Complainer: This nurse is never happy with the plan. Something is always not quite to her liking. She typically would have done things differently. I'm not sure why she didn't go to medical school and do a residency in OB/GYN. Surely she would have been the best.

The Multitasker: This nurse can follow two high risk patients at the same time and will still be the first one to help a coworker when she needs it. She rarely acts overwhelmed and when we see her name on the schedule we are relieved.

Cool as a Cucumber: This nurse will take control of a room that could otherwise fall into chaos. She typically talks in a soothing voice and will look the patient in the eye and succeed in calming her—even in an emergency situation. She will have the same effect on her coworkers.

The Comedian: This nurse should be on stage, as she has some great comedic material that keeps her patients as well as her coworkers laughing. This can be medicinal for a nervous patient as well as an overworked staff. I love working with these nurses!

Control Freak: The nurse that feels the need to control every aspect of her patient's labor, delivery, visitors, monitor, etc. This is exhausting. This nurse typically likes to tell the resident, midwife or even attending what to do. The Control Freak typically likes their patient to be monitored internally. Control Freak nurses are typically control freaks in every aspect of their lives, or at least try to be. Eventually, this does not work for them and things begin to fall apart. Fortunately, the patient rarely notices.

Counting the Days to Retire Nurse: This nurse probably has it down to the hours left. She will typically become a "Bare Minimum Mindy" and do only what she has to do to get to that retirement. Work will become a chore and begin to put a crimp in their lives. That's when they know it is time to retire. This is in no way an insult. It is a right of passage for a job well done. We will all get there. As exciting as the prospect of retiring is, most of them will have a hard time for a while after retirement as they soon realize that labor and delivery is embedded in their soul.

Hall Monitor: This nurse will make sure that the hallway and nurses' station is free from visitors. HIPPA, you know. Family members typically do not like this nurse, but patients do.

Girl Scout: Every room is ready for whatever walks through the door. All paperwork is filled out and ready. The bed cover is turned down, IV is pole ready and taped. We love this nurse!

Her few think-ahead steps are very appreciated when the unexpected walks in the room.

Pigpen: When you go in to take over, this nurse's room has glove wrappers, gobs of lubricant, alcohol swabs, 24 half empty Styrofoam cups half filled with melted ice, wet washcloths, or spoons under the bed. This is not to mention the monitor cords, IV and epidural lines all in a tangled mess. This will send most nurses into orbit and melt down the obsessive-compulsive nurse. This probably has something to do with how she lives her daily life. Although it will drive many of her co-workers crazy, she will still give you all of her attention. She is typically a great nurse.

Coffee Expert: This nurse knows how and when to get the best coffee. Will not settle for anything less than a freshly brewed pot.

Munchausen Nurse: This nurse, even in the most normal situation will predict or find something wrong with all of her patients. She is extremely competent in an emergency, but 90% of the time she typically is a VOD (Voice of Doom).

Granola, "au naturel": This wonderful nurse seems disappointed when her patient asks for an epidural or does not want to walk or be on the birthing ball. She should have been a home-birth attendant, assisting home-birth midwives, as she will walk you through anything. She will talk you out of an epidural better than anyone or happily state "it's too late." You will get through labor and even deem her as your hero. She will most likely have had a natural birth herself. If she can do it, anyone can!

Edward Scissorhands: Magically, everyone's water "accidentally" breaks for this nurse. This is not hard to do on any pelvic exam. This will typically stimulate labor progress whether we are ready or not.

Baby Whisperer: The nurse that comes in after you have done absolutely everything to get your patient delivered for 12 long hours and pushing during the last 3. Before you have even clocked out, she comes out of the room and says, "she's ready" and calls in the delivery team. Grrrr.

Newbie: Deer-in-the-headlights is the best way to describe the new labor nurse. It takes months, even years to develop a feel or become comfortable as a labor nurse. My heart aches for the Newbie, as I remember it oh so well. The tough will survive and it will become embedded in their souls. Typical behavior in the Newbie include: over analysis of the fetal heart tracing, looking for trouble with a magnifying glass—usually convinced they have found something, and calling everyone in for delivery about an hour before it actually happens (which is actually more of a fear of being alone with the patient if she delivers). Don't worry, it eventually will happen to the best of us.

The Beauty (even after a 12-hour shift): I don't know how she does it. Perfectly applied make-up, even after 3 hour of pushing. She manages to find the time to brush her teeth when most of us can't even find the time to pee.

Drama Queen: Her patients are always worse off than the rest of the staff! Her shift was the worst, she had the most trying day and so on. This is not typically isolated to the labor and delivery unit. Drama is her everyday life. It's exhausting.

Nursing from the Desk: This nurse will collect her information from the monitors and not frequent the room as much as she probably should.

Nervous Nelly: It might be because she is a Newbie, but some people are just nervous. Labor & delivery might not be the best match for this type of personality.

C-Section Queen: This nurse seems to be in the OR more than any other nurse. This is typically more of a rut than anything else. This very competent nurse begins to feel as if she is doing something wrong. Eventually, the tide turns and she yet again has more vaginal deliveries.

The Strip Nazi: This nurse watches and critiques everyone else's fetal monitor strip. This may benefit the patient, so it's not necessarily a bad thing, but her manner may be annoying.

Hide and Seek: This nurse conveniently disappears when a new patient walks on the unit. She will also stay well tucked away in her patient's room when all hell breaks loose. The thought of having more than one patient is beyond her. She is the opposite of the Multitasker.

Chronic Call-In-Sick Nurse: She is sick almost more than she's there. Always has a headache and will tend to leave early at every chance she gets. She walks around with an ice pack on her head. This nurse will rarely ever come in to help a busy unit or work more than her required time.

I'm On Break: This nurse will not miss a break or meal and will make sure that someone is covering her. Most L&D nurses will just eat around their patients needs—but not this nurse. She will take breaks as the union contract dictates, no matter what. This is not typically the staff's favorite team player.

The Martyr: This nurse will rarely take a break. Even if offered, she will decline the help. Annoyingly, she will be the first one to complain she did not have a break.

Superstitious Sally: This nurse cringes at the "Q" word (quiet). She won't erase a patient off the board (before computer boards), has special socks to match scrubs, hates working full moons and Friday the 13th, etc. Typically harmless, this quirky nurse is usually fun to work with.

Vaginal Victoria: This nurse will have a vaginal birth no matter what. She knows all the positions and tricks and she's proud! Other staff members are usually in awe of her success rate.

Mother Superior: The labor nurse that has been doing this longer than you've been alive. She's seen everything and usually knows what she is talking about. She seems tough at first, but as you experience your first heart breaking tragedy, and that day will come, she will console and nurture you back to the very competent nurse you are.

Debbie Decel: Everything is a deceleration (drop in baby's heart rate). This is a frequent condition of the Newbie and can be exhausting as it resembles the boy who cried wolf.

These are all pretty good examples of the many personality types you will find on the labor and delivery unit. It is interesting to observe from my perspective, and as I gathered information from others around the country, I realized it is the same everywhere. If you are a labor nurse, I bet you could put names to all of the labels. If you are a patient, it might not be as obvious but could be a fun distraction to label your nurse.

"I'd rather be a stupid person wanting clarification and answers, in order to be wiser, than be a stupid person that blindly believes the lies they are told, without question."

— Shannon L. Alder

HMM...LET'S CLARIFY
CHAPTER 10

I am always in awe when a patient comes to us in labor, terrified, as those they love have showered them with a host of horror stories. Why would anyone do this to someone they care about? I have been witness to hundreds (more like thousands) of births over my 33+ years and can probably count on my fingers the true horror stories I have come to witness. Yes, I realize that it is the patient's perception of the delivery that is most important—but it amazes me that anyone would even get pregnant with some of the scary stories out there.

Have you heard?

You will get paralyzed if you have an epidural.
I have personally never witnessed this. How terrifying to think you may become paralyzed if you choose to manage your pain with an epidural. I would not hesitate to have an epidural. Do you think we want you paralyzed?

First let's explain what an epidural is. Epidural anesthesia is the most popular method of pain relief during labor. More women request an epidural by name than any other method of pain relief. At our institution, the epidural rate is close to 85%. Yes, there have been reported complications and we will discuss them more in an upcoming chapter, but paralysis is extremely rare and personally I have never seen it.

Epidurals increase your risk for forceps or vacuum delivery.
Absolutely not! I will argue this point to anyone who wants to listen. I have had the opportunity, early in my career, to work in a hospital that did not offer epidurals. Barbaric you say? I might agree, but it did teach me a few things. The first lesson I learned is that women will survive labor without an epidural. We were born to do it, and actually do it well. Here's where I disagree with the risk for forceps or vacuums and I am specifically referring to first time moms: When your body reaches that final destination of 10 centimeters, they failed to tell you it could be 2-3 hours of pushing from this point, as the urge to push without the epidural is overwhelming. I still know you can do it, but you will exhaust yourself from pushing for that duration. Now, your sympathetic physician may offer to help end the suffering by assisting the birth with a vacuum or forceps. You agree—anything to end this would be greatly appreciated.

Now, had you had an epidural, the overwhelming urge to push is often from mere pressure, or maybe nothing at all—and you sleep. You sleep only to wake up and have the staff tell you that you are fully dilated and the head is "right there." This will typically result in pushing for under an hour. Most of you will feel pressure when you have a contraction and this is often enough to push well with.

That's my story and I'm sticking to it.

Your water can't be broken for more than 24 hours or you will have a dry birth.
I have been involved with labor and delivery for longer than most of you have been out of diapers and I have yet to see what a dry birth looks like. It sounds horrible, so I am glad I have yet to witness it. I can imagine the concern could be a lack

of lubrication at the time of birth. But let me assure you, when a watermelon delivers through a hole the size of a quarter, there is no amount of lubrication that makes it easy.

As long as the baby is peeing inside you (that's essentially what amniotic fluid is) all will be well.

Prolonged rupture of the membranes is not an uncommon situation. There are typically two risks for prolonged rupture of membranes. The first is potential infection and we can easily minimize your risk by doing fewer pelvic exams and possibly administering prophylactic (preventative) antibiotics. The second potential risk is all that goes along with inductions or augmentations. An induction is when we start from scratch, so to say. You have not begun to change your cervix or contract. Depending on how dilated you are, the methods can be different. An augmentation is kind of a labor boost. This labor has already begun but is progressing slowly. A Pitocin drip is often used and this may statistically increase your chance of a cesarean section, but again, there are many variables.

There are ways to kick-start your labor from home.
If this were true, I think we'd know about it and we wouldn't keep the secret from you. In all my years, there has yet to be a home remedy that will effectively induce your labor. I'm sorry if this disappoints you.

The one thing I do know is that Mother Nature tends to do it best and we don't know what her secret formula is or we would have surely stolen the recipe.

Here are some of the more popular trends utilized in early labor that may or may not make a difference:

Castor oil: Many women swear by this as a way to induce labor, but it should really be avoided. I have actually recommended it in early labor, but with a warning. You will have the worst cramps, followed by pooping your brains out! Your labor nurse may not enjoy this and you will scare your people. The idea is that the castor oil stimulates the bowel,

HMM...LET'S CLARIFY

which in turn stimulates contractions. I have seen it kick early labors into high gear, but it does not look like fun and I have even missed the deliveries. This is not for the squeamish and it is not the time to address your long-standing constipation.

Spicy food: Nurses, especially night nurses, are likely to gag when you barf up your spicy Mexican dinner. They won't let you know they are having a hard time but watch for their tearing eyes. Spicy food won't put you into labor but if you consume it in early labor, it will definitely come back to haunt you and everyone else in the room. It is not wise to eat anything heavy in early labor, as the body will shut down the digestive juices in order to focus on your womanly parts and duties.

A ride in a bumpy car: Good God woman, are you crazy? Doesn't your back not already ache enough? If you are into self-torture and mutilation—go for it, but it is not something that I recommend.

Talk to your baby: Talk to your baby all you want, it won't work. Talk to them when they are teenagers and it still doesn't work. Enough said.

SEX: If feeling like a beached whale with a backache has you in the mood for a roll in the hay, I say go for it. There is something to be said about the release of prostaglandins from semen that may help to ripen the cervix. Here are the issues: 1) Climaxing in late pregnancy is not that easy, but seems to be a factor that improves success. And, 2) Convincing your husband that he won't hurt the baby with his 24-inch penis. (Wink-wink).

Losing your mucous plug means you are going into labor. NOT. I'm not sure who started all this talk about the mucous plug and gave it such notoriety. I have even had women bring in their mucous plugs as if to prove it to me.

At the very beginning of pregnancy some mucus is

accumulated in the uterine cervix generated by the uterus during ovulation. As the mucus thickens, it seals the cervix tightly, blocking the way for any infection from the vagina to the cervix, and thereby protecting the fetus. That's a basic explanation, but you get the point.

It is normal anywhere from 37-42 weeks to pass a mucous discharge that appears very small and clear to something that may look like a jellyfish. It may be a sign that the body is getting ready for labor, but it may just be a result of cervical ripening and dilation that could begin to happen weeks before delivery.

The best advice is to wait until contractions become regular and begin to take your breath away or if your water breaks. Losing your mucous plug, as the only symptom, is not a reason to go to the hospital.

Your Mom did it this way... So will you.
I have had countless mothers of my labor patients convinced that their daughters will labor just as they did. For most, this is just not the case. Do you forget that there is a father who also plays a role in our laboring mom's physical attributes and pelvic structure? I do pay attention to a history of a mother and sisters who have all had cesarean sections, but still opt to adhere to the belief that every woman needs her own trial of labor.

We tend to phase in and out of what we feel to be the best management. But with that said, it is always for the best outcome.

Once a C-section, always a C-section.
No, this is just not the case, but there are exceptions. If you are in a rural hospital that does not have 24-hour anesthesia coverage and a surgery team, then it is likely that a repeat C-section is in order to prevent the risk of a uterine rupture. This is for your safety, because logistically, it would take about an hour to get everyone ready for your emergency C-section. Women with a previously scarred uterus have an

increased risk for uterine rupture in labor. This could be catastrophic to baby and even mom if a surgical team is not in place to expedite delivery. I have witnessed this occurrence more than a few times. Thankfully, our outcomes were good. A note to the labor personnel, even if mom has an epidural, she does have a sense that something is not right before the shit hits the fan. Two of my moms described a tearing sensation in the low abdomen even though they were comfortable with the epidural. So listen to your mothers—they know.

So who is a good candidate for a vaginal birth after a cesarean section? I personally feel it is pretty easy for your obstetrician to help you with this decision. If you had a cesarean section because the baby was breech or had fetal distress, you are an excellent candidate as circumstances failed to give you a fair trial of labor.

If you pushed for three hours, had a 10-pound baby or the baby's head never came down, you'd be much better off scheduling a cesarean section. If this is not what you want to hear, I'm sorry. I do have your best interest in mind, I really do, but babies tend to get bigger after the more you have. If you had trouble squeezing out number one, what makes you think you can push out number two without putting yourself and your baby at risk?

But for those of you who really want a second chance, schedule a repeat cesarean section at or just past your due date. This way, you are likely to go into labor on your own and see how things play out.

All will be well.
There is so much misinformation out there. My coworkers and I often look at each other in disbelief at some of the stories we hear. Many of the things you are afraid of are just not true. Our best advice is not to fall victim to the bad advice, the horror stories and myths. Mother Nature has pretty much got this down. You must trust your body and the caregivers who will get you through this. All will be well.

"Pain is temporary. It may last a minute, or an hour, or a day, or a year, but eventually it will subside and something else will take its place."

—Lance Armstrong

EPIDURAL OR NOT?
CHAPTER 11

I am a fan of epidurals, period. I know I may not be in the majority of midwives, but I love them.

Epidural anesthesia is regional anesthesia that blocks pain in a particular region of the body. The goal of an epidural is to provide analgesia, or pain relief, rather than anesthesia which leads to total lack of feeling. Epidurals block the nerve impulses from the lower spinal segments. This results in decreased sensation in the lower half of the body, which affects women differently. Some have a complete loss of sensation, some are able to move well and still have excellent pain relief, and some may only feel pressure.

Unfortunately, some epidurals don't end up working well. Sometimes the block is only noted on one side and this may or may not be fixed. Often, in the case of a baby that is too big for mom's pelvis (only we don't know it yet), the mom who initially had a good epidural will become uncomfortable again and request many "top-offs." A top-off is a bolus dose of medication given through the epidural catheter that should once again get mom comfortable. An occasional top-off is not unusual as labor progresses, but when she continues to become uncomfortable with minimal labor progress, the writing is on the wall for a potential cesarean section unless we can get that baby to change positions. Labor nurses have a gift when it comes to changing baby positions. The recently infamous peanut ball (literally looks like a giant Mr. Peanut) has helped to rotate many a baby to a better delivery position (occiput posterior to occiput anterior).

Intravenous (IV) fluids will be started before active labor begins, prior to the procedure of placing the epidural. You can expect to receive a liter of IV fluid prior to an epidural. An anesthesiologist, an obstetrician, or nurse-anesthetist will administer your epidural. You will be asked to arch forward and remain still while lying on your left side or sitting up. This position is vital for preventing problems and increasing the epidural effectiveness.

The procedure takes 10-20 minutes and most of it is opening up the sterile kit and getting the medications ready. An antiseptic solution will be used to wipe your mid-back and small area on your back will be injected with a local anesthetic to numb it. This feels like a bee sting or as I tell patients, a pinch and a burn. A needle is then inserted into the numbed area surrounding the spinal cord in the lower back. This is typically not painful but feels more like someone is pressing a thumb to your back with quite a bit of pressure. After that, a small tube or catheter is threaded through the needle into the epidural space. The needle is then carefully removed, leaving the catheter in place to provide medication either through periodic injections or by continuous dosing. The catheter is taped to the back to prevent it from slipping out. Don't worry they will tape it well. Once you are all taped up, you should be much more comfortable within about 10 minutes.

What I Love About Epidurals
I love that the patient gets to sleep through the worst of their labor.

I love that we typically push for less than an hour for a first baby instead of three. (Nurses will agree).

I love that moms are present in the moment, not under the influence of narcotics. I love that I do not have to pull them from another planet to be present during their birth as they are exhausted from the pain and duration.

I love that there is typically very little to repair when the birth is controlled and I can protect the perineum (skin between the vagina and rectum) from tearing or at least, minimize it. I recently was asked by an intern who had watched a few of my "intact" deliveries how I protected the perineum. The trick is when the head looks to be halfway out, a good epidural will let you sit there for a minute or maybe until the next contraction. This is nearly impossible, although I have seen it done, in a woman without an epidural. It is this moment of stretching that saves you from tearing. Epidurals help prevent a vaginal blowout. When pushing is a bit hectic and there is little control due to the intensity, sometimes the baby will exit a bit more rapid than we'd like causing tears in a few different directions. Not to worry though, the vagina is ultra forgiving and heals very well in a short amount of time.

If a C-section is needed, everything is already in place and we can use it (with a bit more medication).

What I Don't Love About Epidurals
There is a common drop in blood pressure that may result in a drop in the baby's heart rate. This rarely results in an emergency, but it can sure scare the parents. I describe it like this: when you go from such an intense state to such a relaxed state in a short period of time, the common drop in blood pressure results in a more relaxed blood flow through the placenta. This may then precipitate a temporary drop in the heart beat or short term decelerations. This typically resolves after a few position changes and a bolus of IV fluids. For the parents to be, this could be a bit scary when 4 people come running into the room to check on their coworker whose patient has a drop in heart rate. Parents, be relieved that everyone is paying close attention.

Moms will not be able to get out of bed or move well without assistance. This is a bit of a bummer to both of us. If the mom-to-be is a bit fluffy, this makes changing positions (which we want them to do frequently) difficult which takes a toll on the nurse's body. Back and shoulder issues are not uncommon among the labor and delivery staff.

The use of a catheter is common in order for the bladder to not become over distended and prevent the baby's head from coming down. If it is not your first baby and things are moving fast, we may be able to avoid this or use a straight catheter which is inserted and removed once the bladder is emptied (a minute or two).

Less than 1% of women who receive an epidural will experience a spinal headache. A spinal headache is caused by the leakage of spinal fluid due to a puncture in the cord. The headache is severe when the patient is sitting up but not while lying down. In some cases, a blood patch may be done. This all sounds terrible (and the headache is) but all will be well very soon without long-term issues.

The Shakes
Some women experience the shakes or shiver shortly after the initiation of the epidural. This typically doesn't last long but is very annoying to the patient and has nothing to do with being cold.

Once an epidural is turned off (typically after delivery), it may take up to two hours to get sensation back into your lower extremities. You won't be jumping into the shower right away.

A small percentage of women will experience mild back discomfort for 2-6 weeks after delivery. This is not enough to even take a Motrin for, but enough to notice.

Some women experience a low-grade fever and the common denominator seems to be the epidural. There isn't much to worry about, but we may see mom and baby's heart rate go up a bit as a normal response to an elevation on body temperature.

No Epidural For You If...
There are some conditions or complications where an epidural

may pose too much of a risk to the patient. This usually has something to do with issues in blood clotting. If you are currently on blood thinners and have not been removed prior to labor, you may not be a candidate for an epidural. The same goes if you have low platelets. There is no magic number, but it will depend on the comfort level of your anesthesiologist. Most anesthesiologist will do an epidural if the platelets are above 100,000.

An active infection including herpes that is anywhere near the epidural site will make it a big fat "no" for an epidural. Remember, it is our job to keep you safe. Spreading an infection to your spinal column will have a potentially horrible outcome. We know you will survive the pain of labor.

If your labor is moving a mile a minute, you will most likely miss your epidural. This does not usually go over well, but I assure you, it will be over so quick and all will be well.

Obesity makes the epidural very difficult to administer. I have actually had doctors tell their patient that they are too fat to get an epidural, but usually it's worth a try. What many people don't understand is the anesthesiologist needs to be able to feel the spaces in your back (between the vertebrae) in order to place the catheter. Excess fat makes this very difficult and it typically takes a bit longer to do. If you are obese, we are not judging you, but please understand that this makes the task much more difficult.

When I am judged by the fact that I do like epidurals, as a midwife, I have to remind myself what the word and true meaning of midwife means, "with woman," and I am. No matter what her choice, I will only give her my opinion if she asks.

"People are giving birth underwater now. They say it's less traumatic for the baby because it's under water. But it's certainly more traumatic for the other people in the pool."

—Elayne Boosler

HUMOR & BEHIND THE SCENES
CHAPTER 12

Don't read this section if you do not have a sense of humor or are easily offended. Shit happens and in any profession you must keep a sense of humor. This is the glue that forms the lifelong bonds between co-workers and creates memories for a lifetime.

I myself, have experienced a mortifying slip of the tongue that sent my coworkers to the floor, probably peeing themselves a bit, while I sit there wishing the moment would just swallow me up and make me disappear.

It was the end of a long and tedious shift. The admissions were endless, my stomach was hungry and my feet were burning. These are the days that you question working a 12.5-hour shift. These are the days you hope you don't mistakenly roll your eyes or groan in front of the next labor patient that rolls through the door.

I still remember this admission like it was yesterday. Room 7, 6:45pm and only 15 minutes to go until my shift was over. I had just admitted this woman for induction having her third baby. If the cervix is still closed or thick, patients will usually come in the night before for a cervical ripening

(Cervidil) before the actual induction that will start 12.5 hours later. So this was the last thing I had left to do—hopefully.

This couple as not your typical "about to have a baby" couple. There was an underlying anger that was palpable and I don't think they looked at each other once during the admission. The husband made a snide remark to his wife that made me wonder how he spoke to her when there was no one around. He was not very pleasant and even threw me an angry glare as I tried to lighten up the atmosphere of the room. How very sad. That poor baby. I am not usually quick to judge, but I did not like this man.

Cervidil actually looks like a white shoelace that contains a small plastic disc at the end. This is the part that contains the medication that we hope will ripen that cervix over the next 12 hours. It is inserted via pelvic exam and the plastic disc is left just behind the cervix. It is relatively painless to insert and we all hope that it causes some menstrual-like cramping or better yet, labor. If not, it is simply removed 12 hours later and Pitocin is started shortly thereafter.

As I sat on the end of her bed, on my very long day, not liking her husband, I said one of the worst things have ever said to a perfect stranger. "Okay, spread your legs and I am going to insert this little plastic dick into your vagina." DICK?!?! I meant DISC! Oh GOD, too late. She slams her legs shut. Behind me, I hear the nurse gasp as she slowly slips out of the room and I can hear her laugh uncontrollably as I sit there hoping to die. I sat there, looked at the patient, wondering how I could possibly begin to fix this. Ugh, I feel sick. I feel the bile that is creeping up to the back of my throat and take a breath. I looked her in the eyes and just plain apologized, not having any good explanation for why I said dick rather than disc. In my head, I concluded that "dick" is what I thought of her husband and that made my tongue divert.

My ever-loving coworkers, to this day, will never ever let me live that one down. I still get nauseous when I think of it.

A milder version of this happened when I triaged a patient and asked her to spread her lips. LIPS?!?! I meant legs. Oh my God, again! She was lovely and started laughing, probably more so at the horrified look on my face. In the end, that was easier to explain. She had the deepest, darkest and perfectly applied lipstick I had ever seen, a sign she may not actually be in labor, something I notice when evaluating patients.

These things don't just happen to me, thankfully. Our labor wing, over many years has compiled a "Nurse Pinhead" compilation of stories that will make you cringe, laugh out loud, and remind you that we are all human!

Cheryl was an amazing night nurse. Loud, animated and downright funny. Unfortunately, the joke was on her this occasion and it would be awhile before she lived this down.

The patient had delivered almost two hours ago prior and was ready to get cleaned up and taken to the mother-baby unit. She was tired from a long labor and had pushed for almost two full hours.

It is not uncommon for moms to pass a bit of blood and maybe even a few blood clots after delivery, especially when it is the first time that the new mother is getting out of bed. It is routine procedure for the nurse to assist the new mom out of bed and to the shower to make sure she is steady on her feet. Occasionally, the new mom may faint or become woozy and unstable. Smelling salts and a wheelchair are typically all that is needed to get her back to bed for a little while longer. She will be fine.

On this particular occasion, Cheryl was running the shower to warm it up while mom was emptying her bladder for the first time since she had delivered. She helped her to the toilet and as mom went to sit down, Cheryl took the bloodied pad from between her legs. As she headed for the garbage with the blood soaked pad, the mom became faint. Cheryl, hoping to prevent a full faint to the floor took the hand that contained the blood soaked pad and attempted to grab the fainting new mom and prevent the fall. Much to Cheryl's horror, the pad, blood clot included, slapped the new mom right in the face! I laugh every time I read this. It's gross but I cannot help it. Needless to say, all turned out fine but Cheryl was now officially dubbed "nurse pinhead."

Nurse pinhead, we have all been there, done that.

All I Can Say Is…Really?

A patient presented to the labor wing and informed the triage nurse that she was "five." "Five" was not specified but the patient was convinced she was in active labor because she was dilated to "five." The nurse asked, "How do you know you are five?" The patient nonchalantly replied, "Because I could fit five fingers in my vagina." This left the nurse speechless and was not quite sure what to do with this information. She left the room shaking her head. She ended up being 2 centimeters, not really in labor and was sent home. We told her it would be best to leave the checking to us.

We only use two fingers and are much less likely to hurt that delicate vaginal tissue. It's the cervix that we are checking. Typically, 1 centimeter is a finger's width, 3 centimeters is two fingers, and so on. The goal is to get to ten centimeters in which we can't feel the cervix anymore. This is commonly referred to as "complete" or "fully dilated."

Morbid Humor

Sometimes things that have gone wrong can make us laugh. Please do not take offense to this next story. I am not making fun or light of any situation, well, maybe my own reaction.

After a cesarean section, the mother will typically recover on the labor wing for a few hours before transferring to the mother-baby unit. As a midwife, I have very little interaction with the scheduled C-sections. The interns will usually assist the attending physician and follow up with post-operative care.

On this particular day, the intern was busy in the operating room and the nurse called me in to evaluate the patient. Her blood pressure was a bit low and as I attempted to assess her, I found her to be unresponsive. The nurse had mistaken her erratic breathing as snoring. I could not arouse her. My mind was racing. As I called the RRT (Rapid Response Team) I looked at her just post-operative belly. Her dressing was dry, her vaginal flow was normal, but as I felt her belly, I could hear fluid sloshing around freely, something similar to the old waterbeds that would just swish back and forth. This is NOT normal! My immediate and correct assessment was that she was bleeding internally and by this point she had bled quite a bit.

Her doctor was fortunately still in the hospital and we had her back to the operating room within minutes. Although I was not part of the operating room team (for which I was thankful for in that moment), the patient had a belly full of blood which when reopened flooded the floor of the OR. She was successfully repaired and put back together. She was transfused with many units of blood products and was suffering from a rare but serious complication of DIC (disseminated intravascular coagulation). DIC is actually a clotting cascade that takes place is the tiny vessels of the body. Blood thinners are needed to turn things around (I know; it doesn't make sense). This results in bleeding in operative as well as non-operative locations. It's not pretty and it's not as easy as just transfusing a pint or two of blood. For this reason, this particular patient was transferred to the ICU for some extra special care.

She was on my mind for the rest of the day and well into the night. As soon as I got through my morning report and rounded on my patients the next day, I took a walk down to the ICU to check in on our patient from the previous day. At the time she was transferred, she remained on a ventilator and I was hoping she was off by now. She would not remember me at all but I thought a friendly hello from the labor wing was in order.

I could tell that she was awake as I approached her room. "That's great," I thought to myself. I walked in and introduced myself. When she replied to me, her speech was slow and purposeful. Oh my gosh I thought, she's damaged! She had the affect of a mentally delayed person. I continued to speak with her for a bit then dragged my devastated ass back up to the labor wing. I was so upset. I ran into her doctor later in the day and expressed my sadness. He looked at me and said, "Cathi, she was always delayed. She's suffered no long term effect that we can see." I didn't know whether to laugh or cry with relief.

When I tell the story now, we laugh. guess it's part of that morbid medical humor that keeps us going. You have to laugh.

"I Can't Push Yet?!"

When I was still a labor and delivery nurse, I had the unusual experience of a mom stop pushing because she had to deliver to a specific phrase of a song. Stunned, but attempting to accommodate, we actually did have her deliver to her favorite phrase thanks to a good epidural and a doctor with a sense of humor. I believe it was an Allman Brothers tune and I wish I could remember the song and phrase. We had to rewind the song a few extra time to get it right, but we did it. I remember mom singing as she pushed. I don't think I have ever loved a song so much that I would consider this, but it definitely was unique for me.

Masturbation in Labor?

Judy was one of our more seasoned labor and delivery nurses. She had many years of experience under her belt and boy did she know her stuff. Judy's only fault was that she could be a bit cranky prior to 9:30am, which I am assuming was her normal wake-up time.

Once report is given, I typically make my rounds to introduce myself to the patients that would be under my care for the day.

Judy and I entered the room together to find the patient masturbating. Her husband was just sitting there as if this were 100% normal. It may have its purpose, but this is not something that I would call normal on the labor wing.

It definitely caught Judy off guard and after we introduced ourselves, we left the room shaking our heads a little bit thinking, now we have seen almost anything. This went on for hours and I'm not sure how she was not sore for weeks after.

The rationale for the patient was that it assisted with pain relief and release. If you do some research, you will find that there is some validity to this. For women who are laboring in the privacy of their own home, this is probably a great suggestion and may help to get through labor.

For a hospital based birth, she must have been very comfortable with her own sexuality to masturbate in front of total strangers in a setting that I would describe as far from intimate.

For Judy, it broke the ice when it came to her first few hours of work. She actually was amazing with this patient.

The Dreaded Mucous Plug
For reasons for which I am unaware there has been an overabundance of attention given to the mucous plug. A mucous plug is literally a plug of very thick mucus lodged in the cervix (the opening of the uterus) that acts as a physical and antibacterial barrier between an unborn baby and the outside world.

As the pregnancy comes to its ripening phase, this barrier will no longer be needed and it will pass vaginally at some point in the weeks, days or hours before labor begins. The mucous plug may or may not be an event. Some women never notice.

On a typical day, our unit secretary is the first person to greet you and take information such as name, doctors name, insurance, etc. This person is not a labor nurse but is extremely essential when it comes to keeping a busy unit flowing smoothly. This, however, is NOT the person to hand your mucous plug to in a baggie. I assure you, it will not go well.

Most labor wing personnel do not care about your

mucous plug, unless maybe you are premature. It has very little to do with onset of labor and is typically not a "problem" that needs to be addressed in the hospital.

It doesn't matter what area of medicine you are in. You think you have seen it all and then something walks around the corner, a brand new experience. I guess that's part of what keep us loving our jobs. My advice is to always keep a sense of humor. It will make your work life much more bearable.

"There are only two ways to live your life. One is as though nothing is a miracle. The other is as though everything is a miracle."

—Albert Einstein

HAPPY ENDINGS
CHAPTER 13

We Were Not Alone

It was late August in 2016, probably one of the more recent and closest events to the publication of this book. It was a crazy, busy summer. The first with our new neonatal intensive care unit which invited a higher risk level of patients. It seemed like every day was more of the same, with no place to put the next patient that walked through the door. Delivered moms being placed in the "holdover area," waiting for a mom that delivered two days prior to leave so she could once again have her private space. Buffalo is turning the corner. Jobs are opening up and the younger generation is staying. More babies are being born and the National Census has not caught on yet. Ask any labor and delivery person, our numbers are up.

Finally, I get to work on a Thursday that is not over capacity with nowhere to go. There are three patients on the board. I can do this; we can actually breathe today. The past two weeks have been hard. Not only did we have a labor wing busting at the seams, but we had two consecutive Thursdays with full-term stillbirths. Ask any nurse, these sad events come in threes and we all hold our breath a bit hoping the next patient is not it.

A call comes from the Emergency Department. They are sending up a very uncomfortable 32-weeker (normal pregnancy is 40 weeks) with severe abdominal pain. There is no time to study and it's too early for us to have her records on hand. Abdominal pain. Preterm labor? Placental abruption? Uterine rupture? Gas?

Well, at least we can get an IV ready and a fetal monitor turned on. Then we heard her—her moans coming from down the hallway. Security informed us that she said she had a history of a ruptured uterus with her last pregnancy. Shit! This was serious and I prayed we had a fetal heartbeat. We struggled to hear anything with the monitor so we turned on the ultrasound and waited for what seemed like forever (it wasn't really). There it was. The baby was alive but his heartbeat was half of what it should have been. The IV was placed and running in fast, within seconds the operating room was made ready.

From the time she rolled through the door to her baby being delivered was barely 15 minutes. Things just seemed to flow without a hitch. What were the odds that her doctor was in the hospital at that time? Well, she was. We had 2 units of blood before we knew her name. Her uterus had ruptured and she was bleeding internally. The baby was bleeding out as well. Upon the first incision, there was an abnormal accumulation of blood that spilled everywhere.

The baby was handed over and no heart rate was heard. Oxygen, intubation and chest compressions (CPR) was immediately initiated. It took almost 10 minutes to get that baby's heart rate to a normal rate.

The most surreal part of this was the calm flow of the operating room. No screaming, no fumbling for supplies. It was as if everything we needed was there in front of us. Everyone knew what to do and when to do it. Typically, when there is an event such as this, we are debriefed at what we could have done better as hindsight is always perfect. But not this time. We all looked at each other in awe and we couldn't think of one thing that could have gone better in this scenario. There was so much more to the room than the human beings within it. I get chills thinking about the experience. We were not alone. Call it what you will, but we had divine help from hands we could not see.

Five more minutes would have resulted in a dead baby and mom would have not fared much better. She was supposed to be at an interview in a rural area. Had this happened there, the outcome for mom and baby would have likely been fatal for both.

Nothing about this event seemed chaotic, even with how serious this was. I know we had help; I know we weren't alone. There was a sense of calm and peace in all of this. Even speaking with her family afterward was peaceful and calm. They were comforting and kind amidst all of this. There was no drama, just peace.

At a week out, the baby was doing far better than expected and did go home with his family about six weeks after delivery. Of course it would be some time before we know if there is any sort of neurological deficit, but with every fiber of my being, I believe that all will be well.

Just prior to publishing this book, I was happy to learn he is doing so well. A miracle for sure.

Later that same day, I admitted a 25-year-old woman with her second baby due in just a few weeks. No fetal heart rate.

Cord Prolapse—ALL ME

It's so easy to judge and blame others as hindsight is priceless and I'm not innocent. But in this case, I am the one you can point fingers at and say I shouldn't have. Lisa was that patient you just fell in love with. She had a go-with-the-flow, easy going personality and would be having her third baby. Piece of cake induction, or so I thought.

I loved everything about her. Her husband was kind and funny and even her very Italian father-in-law would charm me to pieces talking about Italy.

Lisa was sent in for an induction at 39.5 weeks. She was 2-3 centimeters upon admission and had two uncomplicated deliveries prior to this baby. I admitted her at approximately 8:00am on a Thursday morning. She's what I would call a boring patient. She was healthy, no surgery, no allergies. Nada. Not a risk factor to be found. Easy-peasy!

The plan was to start Pitocin, eventually break her water and hopefully have a baby by mid-afternoon. Her history revealed that once her water broke, she went fast. Lisa wanted an epidural so this was a consideration, as I would probably want to break her water after her epidural or just before in order for her to not miss the "window of opportunity." The anesthesiologist on call was probably one of my least favorites. He always took his time in being available to do an epidural and it was obvious we were bothering him. He had no love for obstetrical anesthesia. Although he is not and never would be my favorite, I cannot say anything negative in regards to his skills as an anesthesiologist.

Lisa's doctor wanted me to break her water when I could, in order to expedite her labor. This is a common request by a physician for any induction. Remember, an induction is meant to speed up delivery. Nothing Mother Nature about it. Lisa was becoming uncomfortable with contractions that were 2-3 minutes apart on an infusion of Pitocin. She was now 3-4 centimeters dilated, 80% effaced (thinned out), and -2 station (head engaged in pelvis). I knew that if I broke her water, things would fly. I asked Lisa if she wanted her epidural before I broke her water and she said yes. She was thankful that I would wait to break her water.

A half an hour later, Lisa was comfortable with her epidural when I came in to break her water. Everything should now move along from this point forward at a relatively fast and uneventful pace, or so I thought. I gloved up and did a pelvic exam. There had been no change aside from the fact that Lisa was now comfortable. The nurse opened an amniotic hook for me. It looks obnoxious (like a very long crochet hook) but is actually a very easy and painless way to break water, aka, rupture membranes.

Breaking water is relatively painless and many women initially report a feeling of relief or decreased pressure. It is a warm release of water (amniotic fluid) that generally results in stronger contractions.

I easily ruptured Lisa's membranes and immediately felt something was not right. After a gush of clear fluid, not only did I continue to feel the baby's head, I now felt something else. Was it an ear? No! Shit, I felt a pulse. This told me that I was feeling the umbilical cord. NOT GOOD! When the umbilical cord slips before the head, the head could now compress the cord. This will occlude blood flow to the baby. If the condition is not resolved, the baby will not survive or at the very least will need extensive resuscitation.

I calmly attempted to slip the cord back and prayed this was not happening. I could not. I very calmly told the nurse that I had a cord as not to cause panic in patient or staff. It took her a few seconds to register what I had just said as I tend to remain more than clam in the most intense situations (a gift I am so grateful for). I had an overwhelming sick feeling as I knew they had just taken another patient back for a C-section. Everyone I needed was already occupied. I wanted to throw up.

Within seconds of informing my nurse of our current situation, I had five people in our room expediting our route to the operating room. From the moment I broke Lisa's water, my hand had not left her vagina and would not until my hand meets the surgeons who will facilitate this baby's safe entry to the world via an abdominal incision. I am on the bed with her. My hand is deep inside her keeping the baby's head from compressing the cord that provides life to this unborn baby.

As we were being transported to the operating room, I suddenly felt the baby's fingers grip my hand. I'm not sure how I didn't throw up. But the good news was that the baby was doing well if he could grab my finger. I am so confused, how could a head become a cord, become a hand? I am dying inside as I know, had I not broken her water, none of this would be happening.

Thankfully, the C-section before us had not been started and was put on hold. We were wheeled into the operating room. There were so many voices and the intensity of the situation was suffocating. I was draped under the sterile blue sheets with the patient as my hand cannot let that head compress the cord. At this point, I am forgotten as instruments are hitting me in the head and the operating team is rapidly getting ready for this emergency delivery. My hand can feel the baby's pulse through the cord. A normal heart rate for a baby, as well as this baby, was about 135 beats per minute. Just prior to delivery, I could feel the heart rate slowing to 60's, 50's, 40's and expressed a now panicked urgency to hurry. The hand that reached for mine, was now still.

As I was riding the bed back to the operating room, one of my dearest friends who happens to be an excellent OB/GYN is in the hallway. I knew that she would be able to get that baby out faster than anyone else and begged her to come back and help us get this baby out along with my in-house doctor. She could have said no and probably should have, as obstetrics is one of the highest litigation venues in medicine. I will be forever grateful as she did help us expedite delivery. Dr. Loriann Fraas, YOU ROCK!!!

17 minutes after we had this cord prolapse, a 7 pound 14 ounce baby boy was born. Even though we had every neonatal emergency personnel in place, little Jueseppi (named after his dad), took a big deep breath and cried, even before he fully emerged into our operating room. cried right along with him, silently.

In hindsight, most would say that the baby's head was too high when I ruptured her membranes, and that I shouldn't have. I have witnessed this myself on two other occasions where I had to switch places with the obstetrician so he could scrub for the C-section as I held the head off the cord.

I will fully concede that I was the facilitator to that specific event. I will also say that given that specific exam, 3-4 centimeters, 80% effaced and -2 station, I would rupture membranes again without thinking I would be at risk for a cord prolapse.

Thank God For Epidurals

In my 30 years of obstetrics, I recently had a "wow" moment that I won't ever forget. I doubt the couple involved will forget as well. They were your typical induction, 39+ weeks, 2-3 centimeters dilated and ready to have a baby. Her prior delivery was a set of twins, which she successfully delivered vaginally—not your typical outcome.

A very sweet patient, this 35-year-old, Lucy, was recently divorced and happily engaged to her new fiancé. Her doctor broke her water a short time after she began to have regular contractions on an IV infusion of Pitocin. Her exam was 3 centimeters, 70% thinned out and the head was at a -2 station. She was unsure about an epidural, though she eventually did ask when contractions started to get the best of her.

A short, comfortable while later, I re-examined her and was surprised at what I felt. In all my years of nursing/midwifery, this was a first for me. As is typical, I donned a sterile glove and lubricated with two packets of lubricant (the companies are becoming stingy with the amount of lubricant per packet and if it were my vagina, I want you, the examiner, well lubricated). As I gently inserted my two fingers into her vagina, I was greeted with the very odd sensation of a hand that reached out for mine.

This little baby girl, yet to be out in our world, just grabbed my fingers. My heart melted and ached in the same moment. This was not likely to ever happen again and the odds for a vaginal delivery were not in her favor, only she did not know it yet.

There is a sense of calm that typically comes over me in high alert situations. This was not a crisis. The baby had a strong and healthy heart rate. Mom was very comfortable with an epidural and had no idea that we should be setting up for a cesarean section rather than sitting there so nonchalantly.

In my adrenaline induced ultra calm voice, I told the patient that although it may seem cute, the situation in hand (literally), was not so cute. I informed her that her daughter and I were currently holding hands and this would typically result in an expedited cesarean section delivery. I did not remove my hand from her daughters. I could not believe this woman was going to have a cesarean section after having delivered twins vaginally. This wasn't fair.

Realizing that she was very comfortable with her epidural and baby was doing well, I looked at her and asked if she were comfortable. "Yes," she said. I explained that because she was so comfortable, there was a slight chance that I could try to get her baby girl to pull her arm back up where it belonged.

The irony here was that her mom, a nurse practitioner/lactation consultant, was not in favor of epidurals. I had just explained that I was an advocate for them and gave her many examples why. If it were not for the excellent epidural, my attempt to reduce (or put back) this baby girl's hand would never have been an option. The stars were in her favor today. My attempts to gently push this arm back up would lie between mom's two minute contractions, when things were more relaxed. After 5-6 minutes, all I can feel is the baby girls finger tips alongside her head. This we could deal with. I rolled mom to her right side in hopes that our baby girl would continue to pull her arm back.

I called her doctor and told her she better head this way as the odds for a cesarean section were high and I would prefer she were close.

Two hours later, Lucy was fully dilated, pushed through maybe four contractions, and had one of the more beautiful births that I have been witness to. This was one of the rare moments that went against the odds.

Miracles Do Happen

Throughout history there have been numerous accounts, documentation and stories of miraculous events that warm our hearts and spark our souls to the possibility of the unexplainable.

Most miracles are recognized when the majority of us would have concluded that all hope is lost, although I am sure they happen more than we give them credit for.

The more "rules" we have on what is or is not possible, the less likely we are to be a witness to the miracles that present themselves on a regular basis. Could the Law of Attraction have something to do with it? Better stated as, if you are open to the possibility that anything is possible, are you more likely to witness miracles?

Although I have heard many stories of miraculous recoveries, I have actually had the opportunity to witness a miracle I will never forget.

It was my typical twelve-hour shift as a staff midwife. On the previous night, we admitted a patient I will refer to as Jane, as I was not able to locate her for permission to tell her story. We were inducing for labor. Unfortunately, her story was not your typical admission to the labor wing.

It was determined by early and multiple ultrasounds by different experts in the field that Jane's baby did not have kidneys. The abnormality is called Potter's Syndrome. Potter's Syndrome is a rare condition in which the baby does not develop normal kidneys and as a result, the chances of survival to the due date are not promising. If the baby survives to term (close to the due date) it is unlikely that the infant would survive labor. Kidney function is very important in maintaining adequate amniotic fluid levels that help protect the baby, as well as a multitude of other functions. At best, the prognosis is very poor.

Jane's decision was to carry this baby until it passed or she delivered. Fortunately, our hospital has an outstanding bereavement program to help people in these very difficult situations. Jane's doctor, nurses from the bereavement team, and nursery personnel were all very prepared for Jane's arrival when the time came time to induce labor—amazingly, her baby made it to her due date.

The staff was informed that the baby was likely to die during labor and Jane and her family were also aware of this. Because it would be very traumatic to watch a baby die right in front of our eyes, the decision was made not to monitor the baby during labor.

Here is where the story gets unusual. Jane was admitted at night for an induction. Sometimes the admitting nurse draws an extra vial or two of blood in case there is another test we may want to order. The extra tube was set on the counter. Somewhere during the wee hours of the morning, the vial of blood exploded. In 29 years of working in a hospital, I have never heard of such a thing.

My shift began at 7:00am. Jane was in advanced labor and we all knew it wouldn't be long before she would have to push and deliver what was most likely a lifeless baby. Even with all the preparation, it is so very hard to prepare for this.

Jane's wishes were to hold her baby and no efforts were to be made to revive or resuscitate if she were born alive. Jane pushed well, as her labor was uncomplicated and shortly before noon a very pink, beautiful and crying baby girl was born. Everything seemed so perfect, but we all knew that this baby was going to die in a short period of time based on a confirmed diagnosis by more than one specialist. We bundled that beautiful girl up and handed her to her mother. There was not a dry eye in the room.

About an hour later, Jane asked if she could feed her baby. With nothing to lose and wanting with all our hearts for Jane to make the most of this time, we saw no reason not to feed this baby. The hours went by and this baby was anything but sickly. How could this be? Three separate specialists confirmed this diagnosis. I will add that they are excellent, so an error was not likely.

Eventually we needed to take a look at this child. Here's the miracle. Upon ultrasound, a small kidney was found. When I spoke with her later, Jane was convinced that at the time the tube of blood burst, her baby got a kidney. She went on to say that she had recently lost her grandfather and felt he had a hand in this as well. Jane and her baby were discharged days later and as far as her doctor is aware, years later, the little miracle baby is still beating the odds.

I am honored and feel very blessed to have witnessed this incredible and miraculous birth. I hope each and every one of you may come to witness the awe of being touched by a miracle.

Against All Odds

DeJanese was a beautiful young mom-to-be that I had the pleasure to meet very early in her pregnancy. She was only about 15 weeks along but because she lost a baby at approximately 20 weeks due to an incompetent cervix, she had come in for a procedure known as a cerclage. An incompetent cervix is a cervix that does not stay closed for the entire duration of pregnancy, typically causing a very pre-term delivery of a baby—too early to survive. A cerclage is a type of stitch (like a purse-string) that keeps the pregnancy safe within the uterus. It is typically removed at about 36-37 weeks of pregnancy.

DeJanese had the cerclage placed without any issue. About 3 days later, she arrived to our unit with a complaint of a large gush of fluid. Sadly, I confirmed that, yes, her water had broken and now the cerclage would need to be removed in order for her to deliver this tiny baby that was far from the age of survival. This was so very sad. After she had the cerclage removed, we monitored her on our labor wing, assuming her body would soon go into labor and deliver. Her biggest risk at this point was infection. The barrier between the outer world and the safe inner world was gone.

After some time, DeJanese's body remained quiet and she asked if we could just do nothing. At this point, there was still no sign of infection or impending labor. A brief ultrasound revealed a decent amount of fluid around the baby. DeJanese was sent home praying for a miracle, and so were we.

Her doctor followed her close and kept us updated throughout the remainder of her pregnancy. We were so excited when she hit the 28-week milestone.

The other day, I received a phone call and FaceTime from her doctor. DeJanese, against all odds, had delivered a beautiful 7 pound, 7 ounce baby boy. These are some of the finest moments life has to offer.

Sweet Kristen

It is the end of my very long shift. Not a bad day, just long. I am ready to go see my dad in the assisted living facility around the corner, where every once in awhile I bring him a tiny Jim Beam bottle. I love to watch the reaction of his face when he twists that cap open and smells its nectar. You'd think he was smelling a field of lavender. His face lights up, I see happiness. His alcoholic past has brought him to a life of dementia and a 4 second memory. He is a good dad, and was a good dad. It is so sad that the rest of his life will need to be spent in this place, though a nice place. The people are wonderful. I lie to him every day telling him he is coming back to my house in a week or so. It has been over four years... I'm such a liar but he still loves me so.

Back to Kristen. My shift ends at 7:15pm. It is 6:45pm and a very uncomfortable girl rolls through the labor wing doors. Something is familiar but after 27 years, that is not unusual.

The charge nurse reminds me that this was the girl that lost a baby about 3-4 years ago. It was their first baby. They held that baby for more than 24 hours before they could give it up. If I recall correctly, she wanted to be discharged and taken from the room before we removed the baby. This is never easy but we do try to accommodate in any way we can.

Kristen was rolled into Room 4. The intern was already in checking her. She was 8 centimeters and her water just broke. I knew her doctor lived 40 minutes away and would most likely no make this delivery.

Kristen was calm and sweet to a fault. Amazing for a woman who had been through what she had. She masked the pain ripping through her body in the sweetest way possible, looked me straight in the eye and said, "I would really like an epidural please." The reality of the situation was that it was not a possibility. By the time we had anesthesia in the room, sat her in a very uncomfortable position and washed her back, that baby's head would be working its way out. By the time she got numb, she would have been delivered by ten minutes. Not an easy conversation to have, but the reality of the situation was that there was no time for Kristen to get her epidural.

Dad was standing in the corner, petrified. Could you even imagine his helplessness? Combine this with a traumatic past experience and I'm sure it is almost too much to bear. Unfortunately, there was little time to focus on him.

One of her biggest concerns is that she did not want to tear and therefore need stitches. I told her that because it is not her first baby, we had a great chance of keeping her intact if she followed our voice and did not panic. This is not easy to do without the help of an epidural, but for some reason, she was calm and I knew she would do just fine.

Less than 10 minutes and four contractions later, Kristen gently pushed out a 7 pound, 4 ounce baby boy, perfectly. As far as stitches go, Kristen tore very minimally and actually could have gone without stitches. It has been my experience that just a few stitches to bring tissue together will expedite the healing process tenfold. I gave Kristen the choice. She asked, "What would you do?" I replied, "I would take two tiny sutures." So she did, and within a few moments was feeling so well she could have gone home.

For me, the job comes full circle. The saddest moments eventually see joy. How is it that I get to be there twice? Is it for me or is it for her? Either way, it is a gift and I will take it any day. Life comes full circle.

She was an amazing example of beauty and strength. These are the deliveries that I never want to forget.

In rereading my notes and draft copy for this book, I find it funny how often I refer to deliveries as "the most beautiful," and yet, had I not written anything down, I know I would not remember. This was a very sad realization for me. How many beautiful deliveries am I not remembering? I bet hundreds. But maybe this is not to be my memory, this is one for the family unit that I was made a part of. I am honored.

A recent thank you came in the form of a beautiful family portrait Christmas card. This letter is just one of many that touch our hearts and remind us that what we do counts. This letter was written by Leslie's husband, the first story in this chapter:

Dear Labor and Delivery Staff:

I don't know the names of each individual who was working in your unit on the morning of August 25, 2016, but my wife and I hope that each of them have an opportunity to read this letter.

I am writing this letter to express my sincerest gratitude for the work you perform each day, especially on the day mentioned above. Many people get up every day and head off to what feels like a thankless job. I hope none of you ever feel that way because the work you do is as life changing as any work can be. It is not lost on me that without your effort I could be sitting here today a widower, raising my daughter alone, having lost my wife and son in childbirth. Because of you, my daughter and I are now home with her mom and baby brother. YOU SAVED THEIR LIVES.

This holiday season I want you to know how thankful that I am for all of you and for my family. This little family is whole because of you and for that we are forever grateful. Keep doing what you do. You are great at it. Thank you and God bless you.

Sincerely,
You make a difference in so many lives.

A Minute to Remember

I will leave you with a short scenario that recently choked me up unexpectedly. I easily choke up, but this specific time left an imprint on me and the beauty of the moment was similar to a gong going off in the room.

A local news anchor had arrived in labor during the wee hours of the morning. She had passed her due date and worked right up until she presented to our wing. Her labor went faster than most first time moms, but she was thoroughly enjoying her epidural and able to rest until it was time to push. She was my favorite type of patient. She was not a ball of nerves, she had a go-with-the-flow type attitude and she had a great sense of humor. Her husband, to the contrary, was scared to death. He admittedly stated he did not do well with blood and this holding the leg thing as she pushed was just about maxing out his tolerance. (It was not bloody, by the way.) We had juice in the room and I told him that the first sign that he may pass out would be a sensation of being too warm. I pointed to the chair and instructed him to sit if he had any such sensation.

She was an excellent pusher and did not push long. As the head was almost half out and we knew she was likely to deliver this little one with the next push, her husband looked petrified and I thought we actually might lose him. Although he is not who I typically care about most in this moment, his discomfort was palpable. Before the next and final push, she looked him in the eye and said, "It's okay, we've got this!" He let out a sob in that moment, and I think I did too. Her strength and ability to care about him in one of the most intense moments of her life was one of the more beautiful labor and delivery snapshots that I have been privileged to witness.

"PUSH: Persist Until Something Happens."

—Albert Einstein

TIME TO PUSH
Chapter 14

Don't Forget To Use Your Intuition
We were all born with a God given, gut instinct that will serve us very well if we learn to use it. It is that little voice inside that we should all listen to and trust. It is a form of communication from a much deeper, trustworthy place. It will help us make the best decisions and avoid the worst decisions without hesitation. Decisions we make in a split second are typically the decisions we don't ever regret.

In the world of labor and delivery, I use this gift as often as it will serve me. Most times it serves me, and those in my care, very well.

If you doubt your own gut instinct or intuition, learn more about it and put it into practice. It is one of the most valuable tools you can develop. It will serve you in your love life, as a parent, as a caregiver, and in just about all the life choices that will come your way in this lifetime.

Go Time
So here it is. You are fully dilated and now comes the time to finally push this little one out.

For first time mothers, this can take a while. 1.5-3

hours would not be abnormal. But worry not, you will get there.

For moms without an epidural, the urge to push typically comes just prior to being fully dilated or complete. The urge to push typically wins and there is no such thing as passive descent.

For moms who choose to labor without the epidural and it is not your first baby, pushing will not take long once fully dilated. These are the patients that can fly from 5 centimeters to fully dilated in just a few contractions. Typically, the room should be set up and ready by the time 7-8 centimeters is reached. The obstetricians should be present or well on their way if they want to make this delivery.

The physician or midwife may have a say in the amount or duration of passive descent in individuals with an epidural. Unfortunately, or fortunately, this may be influenced by his or her schedule, dinner plans or desire to sleep.

One of the more notable advantages to pushing without an epidural is that you can push in any position that feels right. Some prefer to push while lying on their side, some prefer squatting, some prefer standing, and the birthing ball is another option.

The experience and comfort level of the labor and delivery nurse will definitely play a role in your position options. The less seasoned nurse will not be so comfortable with pushing in the less traditional positions.

This is the point of focus for all future mothers. It is the event that has consumed most of your thoughts over the past nine months. It is the shortest point of the whole process, and yet the grandest of finales.

For all of us who have been blessed with the ability to have first hands on this new life, know that you have in your own way imprinted the moment and a tiny piece of this new life. I am honored to do such work and am still in awe at every single delivery.

Fads

I have been working labor and delivery long enough to see many practice protocols come in and out of popularity. Inductions and timing, antibiotics, vaginal birth after cesarean section (VBAC) or not, breastfeeding guidelines, and so many more. I make it a point not to become too attached to flavor of the month protocols and remaining open to change. It's really no big deal and actually those of us who have been doing this for a long time actually laugh about it.

I am often stunned that my children survived infancy, as according to today's standards, I did EVERYTHING wrong. I was very young and did not breastfeed for long, I just really did not have a strong desire to do so. If I had been older, there is no doubt I would have breastfed my children, however, I was very young and really did not know better. I have no guilt, it's just how I felt. My children somehow managed to have amazing immune systems, never had an ear infection or asthma, and to my recollection never needed antibiotics. They were off the growth charts the first year of life and then came back down to normal. They did not suffocate because I had bumpers in the crib, or covered them with a blanket. I had one child who preferred to sleep on his stomach and one that slept on her back. Yes, her head was flatter for a spell, but no helmet was needed. They both wore coats in their car seats and used pacifiers for a bit. According to today's standards, I did it all wrong and it is miraculous my children survived. I say this with sarcasm. I look back now and think that the ignorance and go-with-the-flow attitude of my youth was an asset to my child rearing years. I was not stressed about much and all seemed to go well.

Currently the one trend I am not finding humor in is the "baby friendly" status that hospitals are looking to acquire. We currently live in a society that tends to swing like a pendulum from one extreme to another, leaving common sense and balance out of the equation.

"Baby friendly" came to be for good reason and the original intent was good. That would mean less separation time between mom and baby, better breastfeeding success, weight gain for baby, and so on. We have eliminated the traditional nursery setting, much to the dismay of visitors and now leave baby with mom 24/7 unless the baby needed to be placed in the neonatal intensive care unit (NICU). But here is where we get crazy and lose focus of what it is we are trying to accomplish: we completely removed mom's mental and physical status out of the equation.

If you are sleep deprived, do you think rationally? Do you feel well? Do you think you will handle the postpartum hormonal shift well? The absolute answer is no.

Imagine the following scenario. You are a first time mom and are currently on day 2 of an elective induction. Finally in labor, you seem to have stalled at 6 centimeters. Your epidural does not seem to be working as well and you have had many top-offs (a possible sign that this baby's head might not be fitting through your pelvis). An intrauterine pressure catheter (IUPC) has been placed and after 2 more hours, a cesarean section is appropriately indicated after it was noted that you are having strong enough contractions with no cervical change.

You did not sleep well during the Cervidil portion of this induction; you were excited and the bed was anything but comfortable. Your epidural has not given you the best relief. You are tired, but at least the end is in sight and you will soon be holding your little one and maybe able to rest—or so you think. The cesarean section went well and it is now 7:30pm. You are still wrapping your head around the fact you had a C-section and now they are trying to help you get that baby to breastfeed. You have a host of visitors waiting to come in the room and to top it off, you have not eaten in over 24 hours. Mind you, this is a normal, uncomplicated scenario. There was no hemorrhage, no pushing for 2 hours prior to the C-section. There is no fever and the baby is perfect. It is now 10:00pm. All visitors have gone, you had a bite or two and now the adrenaline from the delivery has left your body. You struggle to keep your eyes open, but the incisional discomfort and crying baby do not allow you to drift off into a much needed rest. In the past, your baby would be taken to the nursery so that you may just get a few solid hours of sleep. This is not the case anymore. The baby needs to breastfeed exclusively and pacifiers are frowned upon. This starts the cascade of events that eventually lead to sleep deprivation. Add hormone fluctuations to this and I'm sure postpartum depression rates are on the rise.

We are instructed in our baby friendly (mom unfriendly) classes that we cannot offer to take the baby, but mom has to request it. I find this sad. I would never ask—in fear of being judged as a bad mother.

As labor and maternity personnel we see this. Most of us do see some benefits of not taking baby to the nursery, but we have taken this to the extreme. Thankfully, there are many nurses out there who see that there patients really could use some sleep and will do what she can to help out (without mom having to ask). This is what a good nurse does, she has the interest of the patient a top priority. I encourage moms to speak up. You are the one going home with a new baby which is a bit terrifying in itself, but even worse if you are sleep deprived.

In Closing

It has been an amazing endeavor to write a book that came from my experience, my hands and my heart. Even as I reread this, I am so very grateful that I wrote much of this in the moment as it becomes blurry faster than I'd like to admit.

If you are a mother-to-be, lay person, member of the vital staff, or even an executive producer like the great Dick Wolf, I hope you have learned something new, or at the very least gained some valuable insight and perspective within the wonderful walls of the Labor & Delivery Unit.

A BABY'S PERSPECTIVE, MAYBE

It's so cozy and warm.
I like being upside down.
I love the feel of my cord as it pulsates,
and the sound of your heartbeat in the distance.
The water is warm. I love to swim.
Am I a mermaid?
I love the sound of your voices, Mom and Dad.
Do you feel me kick you? I am right here.
Stop worrying, it will be ok,
all I need is your love and a warm hug.
I am coming to your arms soon.
Mom? I feel your hugs and they are becoming tighter.
There is less room to move around
and I feel I am falling downward.
Mom? Where are we going? What happened to my warm water?
Why do you squeeze so tight? Is Dad hugging us?
Who's touching my head?
It doesn't hurt, but the light is getting brighter and sometimes I feel
like I am holding my breath.
Can we change positions? I feel like I'm being squished.
What is all that noise?
PUSH, PUSH, PUSH.
Mom? Why are they asking you to push harder?
Who's almost there? Who has lots of hair?
Ouch!
My head is in a vice!
Mom, where is my warm water,
that cord that pulsates with a great vibe?
MOM? It's cold.
Why is there so much noise? What's a girl?
OH, thank God they have laid me down on something warm.
I think I can hear your heartbeat; it is familiar to me.
I'm thirsty. Is there food close by?
It has been a long day Mom.
I'm tired and hungry, but we should sleep.
It's a bit scary out here, so hold me close.
I Love you…I love us.

Made in the USA
Columbia, SC
31 March 2025

55971606R00105